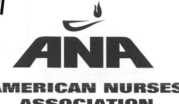

AMERICAN NURSES
ASSOCIATION

GERONTOLOGICAL NURSING:
SCOPE AND STANDARDS
OF PRACTICE

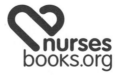

nurses
books.org

AMERICAN NURSES ASSOCIATION
SILVER SPRING, MARYLAND
2010

Library of Congress Cataloging-in-Publication data

American Nurses Association
Gerontological nursing: scope and standards of practice.
    p. ; cm.
Rev. ed. of: Scope and standards of gerontological nursing practice, 2nd edition / ©2001
    Includes bibliographical references and index.
    ISBN-13: 978-1-55810-268-2 (pbk.)
    ISBN-10: 1-55810-265-268-X (pbk.)
        1. Geriatric nursing—Standards—United States.   I. American Nurses Association.
    I. Title. [DNLM: 1. Geriatric Nursing—standards—Practice Guideline.   2. Nursing
    Care—standards —Practice Guideline.   3. Clinical Competence—standards—
    Practice Guideline.   WY 152 A522g 2010]
RC954.A46 2010
610.73′65′021873—dc22   2010046412

The American Nurses Association (ANA) is a national professional association. This ANA publication—*Gerontological Nursing: Scope and Standards of Practice*—reflects the thinking of the nursing profession on various issues and should be reviewed in conjunction with state board of nursing policies and practices. State law, rules, and regulations govern the practice of nursing, while *Gerontological Nursing: Scope and Standards of Practice* guides nurses in the application of their professional skills and responsibilities.

Published by Nursesbooks.org
The Publishing Program of ANA
http://www.Nursesbooks.org/

American Nurses Association
8515 Georgia Avenue, Suite 400
Silver Spring, MD 20910-3492
1-800-274-4ANA
http://www.NursingWorld.org/

The American Nurses Association (ANA) is the only full-service professional organization representing the interests of the nation's 3.1 million registered nurses through its constituent member nurses associations, its organizational affiliates, and the Center for American Nurses. The ANA advances the nursing profession by fostering high standards of nursing practice, promoting the rights of nurses in the workplace, projecting a positive and realistic view of nursing, and by lobbying the Congress and regulatory agencies on health care issues affecting nurses and the public.

Design: Scott Bell, Arlington, VA ~ Freedom by Design, Alexandria, VA ~ Stacy Maguire, Sterling, VA ~ *Copyediting*: Lisa Antony, NC ~ *Proofreading*: Karin van der Tak, Whiteside, NY ~ *Composition*: House of Equations, Inc., Arden, NC ~ *Printing*: Linemark Printing, Upper Marlboro, MD

First printing October 2010.

ISBN-13: 978-1-55810-268-2   SAN: 851-3481   3.5M   10/2010

CONTRIBUTORS

Work Group Members

Barbara McCabe, PhD, APRN, CNS-BC, FNGNA, Co-Chairperson

Barbara Raudonis, PhD, RN, FNGNA, Co-Chairperson

Joanne Alderman, MSN, GCNS, RN-BC, APRN, FNGNA

Wanda Blaser Bonnel, PhD, RN

Jacqueline F. Close, RN, MSN, GCNS-BC

Evelyn G. Duffy DNP, GNP-BC, FAANP

Charlotte Eliopoulos, PhD, ND, MPH, RN

Carmen Galang, DNSc, RN

Debra J. Hain, DNS, APRN, GNP-BC

Melodee Harris, PhD, APN, GNP-BC

Gerilynne (Lynn) M. Jung, MSN, ANP

Gretchen Laubach, BSN, RNBC

Ruth Ludwick, PhD, RN,C, CNS

Liz Macera, PhD, NP-C

Billie Anne Massie, RN,C, BS

Melen R. McBride, PhD, MSN, RN, FGSA

Anita Meehan, MSN, RN, ONC

De Shawn Schmidt, MSN, RN, BC

Dena Jean Sutermaster, RN, MSN, CHPN®

Joyce Varner, DNP, RN, GNP-BC, GCNS

Cheryl L. Waters, RN, MSN

ANA Staff

Carol Bickford, PhD, RN-BC – Content editor

Katherine C. Brewer, MSN, RN – Content editor

Yvonne Daley Humes, MSA – Project coordinator

Maureen E. Cones, Esq. – Legal counsel

Eric Wurzbacher – Project editor

CONTENTS

Scope of Gerontological Nursing Practice

Definition and Description

Gerontological nursing is an evidence-based nursing specialty practice that addresses the unique physiological, psychosocial, developmental, economic, cultural, and spiritual needs related to the process of aging and care of older adults. Gerontological nurses collaborate with older adults and their significant others to promote autonomy, wellness, optimal functioning, comfort, and quality of life from healthy aging to end of life. Gerontological nurses lead interprofessional teams in a holistic, person-centered approach in the specialized care of older adults.

Gerontological nurses are the healthcare professionals consistently responsible for the 24-hour care of older adults across clinical settings. In addition to providing direct care and coordinating services for older adults, gerontological nurses advocate, educate, manage, consult, and conduct research about the dynamic trends, issues, and opportunities related to aging and its effect on older adults. Gerontological nurses have deliberately chosen this title to reflect alignment with *gerontology*, the scientific study of the process and problems of aging, rather than the more limiting branch of medicine known as *geriatrics*, which is concerned with the medical problems and care of the aged.

As early as the 1920s, a few visionary nurses called for the development of gerontological nursing practice because a body of knowledge and skills related to care of older adults across all settings was uniquely distinguishable. Today's healthcare environment—with its increasing focus on aging issues, quality of care, quality of life, access to affordable health care, ethics, and detailed advance directives— is constantly changing.

Various assumptions of aging drive the gerontological nurse's approach and philosophy of care, including:

- Aging is a progressive, irreversible, and natural process that begins at conception.
- All people age differently as a result of genetics and life experiences.
- Older adults can age with high mental and physical function.
- The percentage of older Americans will continue to rise because of changing demographics and increasing life expectancy in the United States.

- Aging encompasses physical, cognitive, emotional, psychological, sociological, and spiritual changes.

- Older adults are a heterogeneous population with varied cultural beliefs and life experiences that contribute to individual well-being and quality of life.

- Older adults seek self-fulfillment and interaction with their environment.

- Older adults are capable of making, and desire to make, informed decisions on how they live and how they die.

- Older adults often experience multiple, interacting, acute, and chronic conditions.

- The older adult's atypical response to many diseases and illnesses often delays prompt diagnosis and treatment.

Readership

Registered nurses, especially those who consider themselves geronto-logical nurses, in every role and setting comprise the primary readership of this professional resource, *Gerontological Nursing: Scope and Standards of Practice* (ANA, 2001). Students, nurse administrators, interprofessional colleagues, agencies, and organizations will find this an invaluable reference. Legislators, regulators, legal counsel, and the judiciary system will also want to examine this nursing specialty scope of practice statement and accompanying standards of practice and professional performance. Last, but not least, the older adults, families, communities, and populations using healthcare and nursing services can use this document to understand better what constitutes gerontological nursing and its members—registered nurses (RNs) and advance practice registered nurses (APRNs).

Today's Context for Gerontological Nursing Practice

It is well documented that the populations of the United States and the world are aging. The number of older adults in the United States will almost double between 2005 and 2030. The baby boomer generation begins to turn 65 years old in 2011 (IOM Report, 2008). The ever-widening diversity of population groups highlights the need for culturally sensitive gerontological nurses.

In addition to the growing numbers of older adults, the oldest-old (including centenarians) are increasing as well. These changing demographic characteristics and the increasing recognition of disability and frailty across the aging spectrum contribute to an unprecedented diversity in the older population. These older adults will have very different needs and preferences related to their care. Technological advances have increased the lifespan of older adults and have contributed to an unprecedented increase in surgical interventions and use of intensive care unit services. Analysis of Medicare data has shown that the significant preponderance of financial expenditures for older adult care occurs in the last six months of life (Hoover, Crystal, Kumar, Sambamoorthi, & Cantor, 2002).

Most older adults live in the community, outside the walls of institutions, and manage their lives relatively independently. A majority of older adults live with at least one chronic condition and rely on healthcare services far more than other segments of the population. Because of their increasing life expectancy, primary (health promotion), secondary (early diagnosis and treatment), and tertiary (restoration and rehabilitation) prevention strategies are appropriate and critical for older adults. However, many myths and stereotypes about aging and older adults exist and interfere with timely, evidence-based quality care to meet the healthcare needs of older adults.

The prevalence of chronic illness increases with an aging population. The development of a chronic illness trajectory provides time for the identification, treatment, and education necessary for adaptation and better living with a chronic condition. Gerontological nurses have the expertise to assist older adults in the self-management of their specific chronic conditions. They can also work with families in identifying the role they can take to partner with older adults to improve their longevity and quality of life.

Evolving models of care for older adults related to living well in the context of having a chronic illness are emerging to meet the diverse needs of an aging population. Systems designed to deliver holistic, person-centered, and coordinated care are now available and continue to be developed specifically for older adults. Community-based housing options and related services enable many older adults to remain in their homes or relocate to group-type housing. The traditional setting of long-term care is slowly changing.

Although Medicare has expanded its coverage to some preventive services, such as screenings for specific cancers, some vaccinations, bone density screening, and diabetes monitoring, many gaps in coverage remain. Medicare does not pay for hearing aids. Dental care is not covered despite growing evidence that oral health has a direct impact on overall health. Medicare's acute care focus persists, although the healthcare needs of the majority of its policy holders are related to chronic illnesses.

Family caregivers are an integral part of community-based care for the aging population. Many of these individuals assume the role of care provider without the benefit of formal and informal healthcare education. Family caregivers provide much-needed care and support to older individuals, and at the same time balance full-time employment, often with child care responsibilities. They fill in the gaps that exist in today's healthcare delivery system. In many instances, family caregivers neglect their own health and jeopardize their financial stability by paying out of their own pockets for services, supplies, and medications not covered by insurance.

History and Evolution of Gerontological Nursing as a Specialty Practice

In 1906, the first article addressing care of the aged was published in *American Journal of Nursing*. Historically, care of older adults had been delegated to the nursing profession and not to medicine.

Lowering the cost of caring and maintaining sick older adults had its beginnings with Florence Nightingale and Agnes Jones during the 1800s in England. Consider that in the early 1900s, life expectancy was about 47 years. During this time, care was provided by family members. From 1800 to the 1930s, almshouses were a norm of care for various groups of poor people. They experienced separation from society and were placed in areas considered to meet common issues; i.e., asylums for the insane, jails for criminals, and foster homes for children. It was during this time that Lavinia Dock, a nurse, and Carolyn Crane, a social activist, found themselves attending to the chronically ill who were elderly. In 1912, the American Nurses Association Board of Directors created a committee to supervise nursing services in almshouses. The World War I era of 1910 to1920 included efforts at improving nursing services at almshouses. In 1925, *American Journal of Nursing* ran an article that "called for nurses to consider a specialty in nursing care of the aged" (Ebersole and Touhy, 2006).

During the 1930s, almshouses became nursing homes and, with the passing of the Social Security Act in 1935, an elderly individual was able to purchase care with these funds. There was no regulation of care, and the number of professional nurses was low. However, this changed in the 1940s, when public health nurses conducted inspections, identified deficiencies, and made evaluations public. There was emphasis on rehabilitation of the elderly. Nursing homes were thriving in the 1950s, and the Kerr-Mills Medical Assistance to the Aged Act provided direct payment to care providers. In 1950, the first book on nursing care of older adults was written by Newton and Anderson. In 1952, the first research article was published on chronic disease and the elderly in the generic issue of *Nursing Research*.

Numerous policy changes occurred during the 1960s and1970s, in part as a result of increased government involvement, research, and the growing numbers of older adults. By 1961, 15 million Americans were older than 65, and life expectancy was approaching 70 and beyond. In 1965, the Medicare and Medicaid program began and the Older Americans Act became a cornerstone to improve the quality of life for older adults. At Duke University School of Nursing, Virginia Stone (1966) developed the first master's degree program in gerontological nursing specific to the role of clinical nurse specialists. With federal funding from the U.S. Department of Health, Education and Welfare, the 1970s brought about the expansion of programs in nursing schools for gerontological nurse practitioners (NPs) and gerontological clinical nurse specialists (CNSs) that focused on care of the elderly.

Late in the 1980s, nursing research showed that improved care of the older adult can be achieved and should be an appropriate expectation within the nursing profession. Infusion of evidence-based practice in the clinical care of older adults is a vital component in nursing education and in all healthcare facilities. Some key events in gerontological nursing of the last four decades are highlighted in the chronology in Figure 1.

The continuing need for more registered nurses and advanced practice nurses who have included or attained certification in gerontological

1976　ANA renames its Geriatric Division the Gerontological Division to reflect a health promotion emphasis; ANA publishes the first document on Standards for Gerontological Nursing Practice.

1977　USDHHS, Bureau of Health Professions, Division of Nursing, provides funding for the first gerontological nursing track at the University of Kansas School of Nursing under Sr. Rose Therese Bahr's leadership.

1981　ANA Division of Gerontological Nursing issues statement regarding Scope of Practice.

1984　National Gerontological Nurses Association's (NGNA) Division of Gerontological Nursing Practice becomes Council on Gerontological Nursing.

1990　ANA establishes a division of Long-Term Care within the Council of Gerontological Nursing.

1993　National Institute of Nursing Research established as separate entity, opening opportunities for research on care of older adults.

2000　ANA publishes *Scope and Standards of Gerontological Nursing Practice.*

2000　American Association of Colleges of Nursing (AACN) and the John A. Hartford Foundation Institute for Geriatric Nursing publish recommendation for baccalaureate competencies and curricular guidelines in geriatric nursing care.

2004　AACN and the Hartford Geriatric Nursing Initiative (HGNI) publish the Nurse Practitioner and Clinical Nurse Specialist Competencies for Older Adult Care.

2008　ANA convenes a panel of gerontological nurse experts to review and revise the existing *Scope and Standards of Gerontological Nursing Practice* (2000).

2010　*Gerontological Nursing: Scope and Standards of Practice* is published.

Figure 1. Chronology of Gerontological Nursing Practice, 1976–2010

nursing remains a reality as we move into the second decade of the 21st century. Several entities have provided funding and support to increase the availability of gerontological nursing education through formal academic education or continuing education and certification programs.

Practice Settings for Gerontological Nursing

Whatever the setting, gerontological nursing is a person-centered approach to promoting healthy aging and the achievement of well-being. It enables the person and their caregivers to adapt to health and life changes and to face ongoing health challenges (Kelly et al 2005). Eliopoulos (2010, p. x) has stated, "... that if done properly, gerontological nursing is among the most complex, dynamic specialties nurses could select. To practice this specialty effectively, nurses need to have a sound base in gerontology and geriatric care, an appreciation for the richness of unique life experiences, and the wisdom to understand that true healing comes from sources that exceed medications and procedures."

The goal of gerontological nursing care is to help older adults function as fully as possible by realizing their highest potential. Collaboration with older adults promotes well-being and the optimization of functional abilities. The gerontological nurse may need to engage in a strong advocacy role when supporting the older adult in such events as making end-of-life decisions; wishing to age in place and not be displaced from familiar surroundings; and escaping from abuse, neglect, or exploitation from family, friends, or others. Research findings are incorporated through the application of theory and evidence-based nursing therapeutics to meet the older adult's goals and expected outcomes (Capezuti, Zwicker, Mezey, & Fulmer, 2008). Gerontological nurses care for older adults in a variety of practice settings: home, acute care, short- and long-term nursing facilities, and community-based programs.

Many healthcare facilities that have become specializezd centers focusing on care and treatment of cancer and cardiovascular disease benefit from a strong gerontological nursing presence. Private and group practices employ gerontological nurses who oversee the health care of their designated panel of older adults and consult with colleagues as needed for others. Gerontological nurses play a significant role in identifying and establishing healthcare services for the often hidden and very vulnerable older adults living on the street, in homeless shelters, and corrections facilities. Gerontological nurses are also present in faith-based communities, assisted living and group home settings, and Alzheimer and dementia care facilities.

Gerontological nurses may combine practice with academics in faculty positions in nursing, medical, and other health professional schools. They may play non-clinical roles in the planning, policy, and operations sectors of government programs, community organizations or agencies, or research centers. Gerontological nurses may choose to continue their advocacy initiatives through election or appointment to public office in local, state, or national legislative or regulatory bodies, including those entities that provide emergency preparedness and disaster response. International organizations and agencies are addressing the world's aging population and need gerontological nurses to inform discussions and direct and staff the associated initiatives.

Gerontological nurses in every setting use the nursing process as the essential methodology by which the older adult's goals are identified and achieved. The nursing process comprises assessment, diagnosis, outcomes identification, planning, implementation, and evaluation. Additionally, coordination of care has been shown to be essential. The accompanying standards of gerontological nursing practice and the associated measurement criteria provide a detailed description of these nursing activities.

Education of the Gerontological Nurse

The Institute of Medicine's 2008 report, *Retooling for an Aging America: Building the Health Care Workforce*, includes the dire prediction of a scarcity of all types of adequately prepared healthcare workers to care for the growing population of older adults. This includes a scarcity of registered nurses even minimally prepared to meet the preferences and needs of an aging population. There is an acute shortage of nurses choosing to specialize in gerontological nursing; less than 1% of the registered nurses in the United States are certified in gerontological nursing (Stierle et al., 2006).

Studies show that adults 65 years and older represent almost 50% of all admissions to hospitals. Consequently, many hospitals recognize that their nurses need the specialty knowledge of gerontological nursing in order to meet the needs of their older adult patients (Stierle et al., 2006). In order to meet The Joint Commission (TJC) criteria on patient safety, nurses working in accredited hospitals need to embrace the knowledge and skills required to identify geriatric syndromes and know-how to prevent iatrogenic complications. The older adult often presents at admission with numerous chronic illnesses and multiple medications, sometimes described as polypharmacy. Because the older adult is physiologically more susceptible to drug interactions, the gerontological nurse's recognition of subtle signs and symptoms can avoid an iatrogenic episode. The gerontological nurse's astute assessment helps older adults to avoid circumstances that compromise their health, safety, and well-being.

Many, but not all, schools of nursing have gerontological nursing courses in their undergraduate nursing curricula. One of the barriers to the development of such courses is the lack of faculty prepared in gerontological nursing. Recognizing this critical need, the John A. Hartford Foundation funded the Geriatric Nursing Education Consortium (GNEC), a national initiative of the American Association of Colleges of Nurses (AACN) and the Hartford Institute for Geriatric Nursing. The goal of this initiative is to educate nursing faculty in the fundamentals of gerontological nursing and the use of gerontological curriculum resources. The Hartford Foundation also funded the Geropsychiatric Nursing Collaborative to enhance the knowledge and skills of nursing to provide improved mental health care to older adults.

Distance education incorporates the rapid advances in communications technology to provide students, and practicing registered nurses, access to degree offerings and continuing education programs in gerontological nursing. Because the Internet and the World Wide Web are also sources of information for older adults and their families, the gerontological nurse must be prepared to guide older adults, family members, and caregivers in the skillful, informed, and effective use of these resources.

History of Gerontological Nursing Education

Although in roughly the same time frame, the development of the education of entry-level and advanced-level gerontological nurses have been distinct enough to merit their own summary.

Entry Level: The structured inclusion of gerontological nursing content in the undergraduate nursing curriculum can be summarized as follows:

> *Early 1960s:* The first standards for gerontological nursing practice were developed by the ANA Gerontology Division. ANA certification for gerontology nurses as generalists followed, and much later, certification was provided to CNSs and NPs with master's and doctoral education in gerontology. These activities were greatly influenced by the establishment of Medicare and Medicaid in the Social Security Act, Titles 18 and 19, and continue to be a significant influence on gerontological nursing education.

> *1981:* The Robert Wood Johnson Teaching Nursing Home Programs and the Kellogg Foundation supported a national focus on quality long-term care by linking nursing homes with academic nursing programs.

> *1990:* The John Hartford Foundation committed long-range support for curriculum reform and development of academic centers of excellence.

The integration in the undergraduate curriculum of gerontology content and mental health and psychiatric content has occurred in various ways:

• Prenursing requirement of a communications course;

• Clinical placements in long-term care settings; and

• Collaborative teaching of faculty in adult care and in psychiatric nursing.

This blending continues to be a dynamic process, with the end goal of creating a generalist gerontological nurse who has strong knowledge and skills in the care of older adults. In 2009, 63 programs prepared baccalaureate graduates for gerontological nursing practice.

Graduate Level: Advanced preparation in gerontological nursing evolved:

> *1966:* The first master's degree as a clinical nurse specialist was offered at Duke University, and the first master's degree as a gerontological nurse practitioner at the University of Massachusetts Lowell.

> *1970s:* Gerontological mental health, currently known as geropsychiatric nursing, was added as a subspecialty to psychiatric

nursing. The degree was intended for clinical nurse specialists in long-term care and was later adapted for students in the NP programs for the family, adult, and gerontology specialties.

Over time, the trend of blending curricula led to the present category of nurses with master's degrees required for the role of the advanced practice registered nurse. APRNs include certified nurse specialists, nurse practitioners, certified nurse midwives, and certified registered nurse anesthetists. Some of these nurses pursue doctoral degrees in nursing or in other fields. Although doctoral programs in nursing existed in the 1950s and 1960s, the emphasis on the science of nursing and the clinical practice of nursing developed much later, as summarized below.

1980s: National Institute of Mental Health (NIMH) supported minority nurses through the American Nurses Association, and some trainees focused on geropsychiatric nursing.

1990: NIMH supported training for nurses in academic and clinical doctoral programs in geropsychiatric nursing.

1996: An infusion of support for pre- and postdoctoral education in gerontological nursing created Centers of Gerontological Nursing Excellence (http://www.gerontologicalnursing.info/; www.hartfordign.org).

2000: The John A. Hartford Foundation's program, Building Academic Gerontology Nursing Capacity (BAGNC), began (http://www.hgni.org/).

2004: Atlantic Philanthropies committed its resources to postdoctoral fellowships in gerontology nursing.

Basic Nursing Education and Gerontological Nursing

Gerontological nurses require a skill set that includes knowledge of normal aging, common disorders, and usual and atypical presentations of illness. Content in gerontological nursing is needed in all nursing programs, from entry-level to advanced practice programs. While not all nurses will consider themselves gerontological nurses, almost all nurses will encounter older adults in their practice. Nurses require the knowledge and skills to assist older adults in a broad range of nursing care issues, from maintaining health and preventing illnesses, to managing complex, overlapping chronic conditions and progressive/protracted frailty in physical and mental functions, to palliative care. Basic competence is critical to ensure the best possible care for diverse populations of older adults.

The entry-level nursing curriculum is intended to prepare professionals for general practice. Although specialization in the care of older adults is relegated to the graduate-level curriculum, gerontology content is introduced in undergraduate programs in various ways. Some nursing programs integrate knowledge and skills throughout the curriculum; others have a stand-alone course in gerontological nursing. A combination of these approaches may be best studied through reporting of outcomes and numbers of graduates who become certified in the specialty of gerontological nursing.

Essential educational competencies and academic standards for care of older adults have been developed by national organizations such as the American Association of Colleges of Nursing (AACN) for both basic and advanced nursing education. AACN has identified 30 educational undergraduate competencies for care of older adults and 47 educational competencies for advanced practice graduates (http://www.aacn.nche. edu/Education/gercomp.htm). Despite these lists of competencies, however, there remains a lack of consistency among nursing schools in helping students gain needed gerontological nursing information and skills. AACN has recommended focus on faculty expertise, including gerontological nursing in the curriculum, enhancing educational opportunities with technology, cultivating partnerships to promote education in gerontology, and implementing strategies to increase student interest in gerontological nursing careers.

Graduate Nursing Education and Gerontological Nursing

Educational preparation is needed for both the care of older individuals and the care of populations of older adults. Graduate programs in recent years have focused on preparing the gerontological NP and gerontological CNS for advanced practice nursing and the leadership required to be advocates for care of older adults. There are also opportunities for practice specialties such as geropsychiatric nursing, ethnogeriatric nursing, and global/international gerontological nursing. Advanced practice nurses are needed for educational and leadership roles as well; however, challenges exist in attaining the number of graduates to meet these needs. In doctoral programs across the country, specializations in gerontological or geropsychiatric nursing and gerontological nursing research are options available to students. Opportunities for pre- and postdoctoral specialization exist.

According to the Consensus Model for APRN Regulation: Licensure, Accreditation, Certification and Education (2008), "the education, certification, and licensure of an individual must be congruent in terms of role and population foci. APRNs may specialize but they cannot be licensed solely within a specialty area. APRNs are educated in one of four roles; one of these is the adult-gerontology nurse practitioner. The population focus, adult-gerontology, encompasses the young adult to the older adult, including the frail elderly. APRNs educated and certified in the adult-gerontology population are educated and certified across both areas of practice and will be titled Adult-Gerontology Certified Nurse Practitioner (CNP) or Clinical Nurse Specialist (CNS). Therefore, the education program should include didactic and clinical education experiences necessary to prepare APRNs with these enhanced skills and knowledge." A target date for full implementation of the Regulatory Model is the year 2015. The document is available at http://www.aacn .nche.edu/education/pdf/APRNReport.pdf.

Gerontological Nursing Clinical Education Opportunities across Diverse Settings

Student clinical education opportunities serve as a prelude to practice and are integral to gerontological nurse preparation. Students should be expected to interact with older adults across all healthcare settings. While debate exists about what clinical settings are best for student learning, particularly for beginning students, there is support for learning experiences that involve healthy older adults. In addition, varied experiences across a continuum of care in acute, long-term, home, community, and primary care settings offer many positive teaching and learning opportunities.

Underutilized settings include long-term care, primary care, home, and community-based services. Long-term care, which includes a wide variety of services (e.g., nursing homes, assisted living, adult day health, programs of all-inclusive care), offers rich opportunities for clinical experiences that help students understand the care (health, illness, economics, personal, and social) of older adults who have a disability or one or more chronic illnesses. Primary care settings, (e.g., clinics, offices) help students develop insight into the health and illness issues that older adults and their families regularly face. Meeting older adults in their homes provides rich student learning opportunities about the requisite adaptations for aging in place. Thus, an important focus for the clinical component in gerontological nursing education is a continuum of clinical care experiences that combine theory, science, and clinical practice grounded in reality.

Ongoing Professional Development

Because fewer than 1% of the 3.1 million nurses in the United States are certified in gerontological nursing, the need for staff training and continuing education programs focused on the care of older adults is one of the priorities for the Hartford Institute for Geriatric Nursing (www.consultGeriRN.org). Evidence-based clinical resources and online continuing education modules are available at this clinical web site. For example, a four-module curriculum on the care of older adults was developed specifically to guide the RN who wishes to become certified as a generalist; it includes a program for the certified advance practice registered nurse in gerontological nursing.

An earlier approach to gerontological nursing competence was the Nurse Competency on Aging (NCA) project. In 2002, the project was launched to increase the knowledge and skills of registered nurses in specialty areas to deliver appropriate and science-based care to older adults. The Atlantic Philanthropies (USA) funded a five-year initiative awarded to the American Nurses Association (ANA) through the American Nurses Foundation (ANF). It represented a strategic alliance among ANA, the American Nurses Credentialing Center (ANCC), and The Hartford Institute for Geriatric Nursing. The goals were to: a) enhance geriatric activities of national specialty nursing associations; b) promote gerontological nursing certification; and c) provide a web-based comprehensive geriatric nursing resource center (Mezey, Stierle, Huba, & Esterson, 2007).

Building on the work of the NCA project, the Hartford Institute for Geriatric Nursing is supporting the Resourcefully Enhancing Aging in Specialty Nursing (REASN) project to move to a new and higher level of engagement in geriatric care. The overall goal of the REASN project is to deepen the involvement of specialty nursing associations in improving nursing competencies in providing optimal care to older adults (Hartford Institute for Geriatric Nursing, http://www.consultgerirn.org/specialty_practice/REASN/).

In 1988, concerns over the interplay among cultural beliefs, health, and aging issues, particularly among ethnic and racial minorities and immigrant older adults, led to the development of ethnogeriatric curricula and educational resources under the U.S. Health Resources and Services Administration (HRSA) initlative to establish Geriatric Education Centers (GECs) across the United States. A core curriculum created by a collaborative of 34 HRSA-funded GECs was disseminated widely to nursing and other health disciplines (www.stanford.edu/group/ethnoger). A postgraduate fellowship in ethnogeriatrics enabled nurse educators, nurses at the pre- and postdoctoral levels, and advance practice nurses to infuse the acquired knowledge and skills into their roles and responsibilities (www.sgec.stanford.edu). Ethnogeriatrics serves to enhance the education, research, and practice of transcultural nursing, particularly in regard to the national goal of eliminating health disparities.

Older adults with mental health disorders are experiencing greater longevity (Crystal, Sambamoorghi, Walkup, & Akincigil, 2003). Most mental health conditions in older adults are undiagnosed and untreated. There is a shortage of expert gerontological nurses across all settings to care for older adults with anxiety, depression, illicit prescription drug use, alcohol abuse, post-traumatic stress disorder, elder mistreatment, delirium, and the dementias. The growing recognition of older adults with mental health conditions has brought about changes in gerontological nursing education, practice, and research.

Historically, several models for geropsychiatric nursing have been suggested to address the needs of older adults with mental health conditions. In the 1970s, the addition of two subspecialties in psychiatric nursing was brought about by the awareness in the rise of substance abuse and addiction and the unmet mental health needs for older adults (Morris & Mentes, 2006). In 1977, the term "geropsychiatric nursing" first appeared as a subject category in the Cumulative Index to Nursing and Allied Health Literature (Bunside, 1981). Geropsychiatric nursing in the 1980s focused on the clinical nurse specialist role and long-term care (Morris & Mentes, 2006). In 1981, Burnside devoted nine chapters to Mental Health: Theory and Therapy in the second edition of her book, *Nursing the Aged*. In 1990, the literature focused upon education for geropsychiatric nursing for undergraduate and graduate nursing students. At the graduate level, content in geropsychiatric nursing was emphasized in a variety of advanced practice nursing specialties (Morris, & Mentes, 2006). There were recommendations for blending the gerontological nursing specialist and the psychiatric-mental health nurse specialist and, more recently, blending the NP and CNS roles that focus on older adults (Morris & Mentes, 2006). Graduate programs in geropsychiatric nursing were also developed. Currently, there is no certification in geropsychiatric nursing at the advanced practice level.

In recent years, geropsychiatric nursing has experienced a rapid transformation.The scope of practice of geropsychiatric nursing that was once defined by a specific age has reconceptualized the definition of aging to include the last decades of life (Butcher, 2006). This transition away from a medical model allows gerontological nursing to reflect a more interdisciplinary approach that addresses disease process as well as health promotion and healthy, successful aging (Butcher, 2006). The future vision of geropsychiatric nursing includes integrating the mental health conditions of older adults into continuing education and nursing curricula. Translational and interdisciplinary research is also needed to address end-of-life, genetics, family care giving, mental health promotion, and mental health conditions in the later decades of life (Kolanowski & Piven, 2006; Puentes, Buckwalter, & Evans, 2006).

Faculty preparation in gerontological nursing varies from self-education to formal graduate education, including doctoral and postdoctoral studies. The latter may include a stand-alone training through a fellowship program, particularly when the trainee is pursuing a mid-career change. The AACN offered regional faculty development training programs from 2007 to 2009 through the Geriatric Nursing Education Consortium (GNEC), with support from the John Hartford Foundation. The goal is to cultivate faculty who would enhance undergraduate curricula by integrating gerontology/geriatric knowledge and positive attitudes about aging and establish programs of research in gerontological nursing.

Educators in academic and nonacademic settings who teach aging content may develop, teach, and evaluate a gerontology curriculum based on nationally developed competency standards and according to the learning needs of target learners and institutional goals. To date there is no formal professional gerontology certification specifically for nurse educators. National data are not available on the number of academic nurse faculty and nonacademic nurse educators who teach content about care of the older adult, their educational preparation, or their influence on learners' career choice to specialize in gerontological nursing or build a nursing research program in the field.

Gerontological Nursing Competencies and Certifications

The Institute of Medicine (IOM) recognizes the current, increasing shortage of professionals with gerontological and geriatrics expertise. Models have been tested and proposed to address this shortage through infusion of gerontology content into other practice specialties. Additionally, the IOM urges that efforts focus on increasing the number of professionals educated in gerontology (IOM, 2008). The need for a competency focus in gerontology can be addressed through a certification process that provides the opportunity to demonstrate and gain acknowledgement for competency. *Nursing: Scope and Standards of Practice* (ANA, 2004) documents nursing applications that include age-appropriate and culturally sensitive care. Specific criteria that direct competent care for older adults across healthcare settings have been published.

Certifications in gerontological nursing for both registered nurses and advanced practice registered nurses (APRNs) are available and should be included in every gerontological nurse's professional goals.

Basic Certification: This category of certification exists for RNs who work primarily with older adults and wish to demonstrate their competence in assessing, managing, implementing, and evaluating health care to meet older adults' specialized needs.

Advanced Certification: This certification is for NPs and CNSs who graduated from appropriately designated programs that teach advanced gerontological nursing care to older adults. As designated by certification, these APRNs demonstrate expertise in providing, directing, and influencing the care of older adults and their families.

In response to the increasing need for APRN gerontological nursing practice and leadership, the Gerontological Nurse Practitioner Alternate Eligibility Examination was recently developed (ANCC, 2008). This alternate certification examination permits individuals who are educationally prepared as adult, family, or acute care NPs to specialize and become certified in the advanced practice of gerontological nursing.

Additional Issues in Gerontological Nursing Education

Issues that merit further consideration in gerontological nursing education include those described below.

Shortages of faculty to teach content related to older adults. Especially with the aging population and general nursing shortage, more faculty numbers are needed to prepare students to provide quality care for older adults.

Best practices in gerontological education. The need for further research is extensive and includes identifying effective strategies to: generate interest in care of the older adult, motivate students to pursue gerontological nursing careers, systematically assess best teaching methods to establish gerontological competencies at the undergraduate level, and examine the use of simulated clinical experiences.

Education about care of older adults for unlicensed assistive personnel under nursing supervision. Issues include not only education of nursing assistants, but the need for further education of new professional nurses in their supervisory roles. As supervisors, gerontological nurses need to know, for example, the supervisory roles, including the roles of delegator and coach; regulations and guides for direct care staff practice; and focus on a positive work environment to retain paraprofessional staff. Strategies to recognize their contributions and opportunities for educational updates and continued education are needed (IOM, 2008).

Ongoing education/continuing education. As noted, education is needed for both paraprofessional and professional staff. Newer movements focusing on culture change in the long-term care setting may affect the education of staff as well. Furthermore, the current shortage of professional nurses, particularly those with gerontological nursing preparation, and the projection that the shortage will become more severe have led to an increase in the number of non-U.S.-educated nurses who are aggressively recruited by representatives of the U.S. healthcare system. Mixed into this healthcare pool are physicians from other countries who received nursing degrees and are licensed registered nurses in the United States.

Recently, the number of registered nurses from other countries reached 14% of nurses in the United States, compared to 10% in 1995 (Brush, 2008). Many are employed in long-term care settings, and often their training in care of older adults is developed and provided by their employers. National standards for gerontology training curricula for foreign-educated RNs are yet to be developed. As they find employment in other types of healthcare settings and deliver care to older adults, staff education and continuing programs will be critical resources to assure that they develop, maintain, and refine their knowledge and skills in gerontological nursing.

Gerontological education for informal caregivers. Students need skills to prepare families as informal caregivers. It is important that students and graduates appreciate that caregiver education is important, educator skills are necessary, and knowledge about caregiver resources and tools is essential.

Technology and gerontological nursing education. There are benefits to the technologies to enhance clinical practice and in providing ongoing education. Personal digital assistants (PDAs), academic/electronic health records (AHR/EHR), web resources, simulations, and other technologies can provide easy access to best-practice evidence for the clinician. This enables immediate care decisions and provides evidence-based practice guidelines for education to older adults and caregivers. Additionally, faculty need to be aware of diverse informatics competencies (NLN, 2008) and tools that can help promote safe quality patient care. The Technology Informatics Guiding Educational Reform (TIGER) initiative is led by nurses to establish guidelines for organizations to follow as they integrate informatics into practice and academic settings (https://www .tigersummit.com/Home_Page.html).

Sample Resources for Gerontological Nursing Education

The Hartford Institute of Geriatric Nursing (HIGN), in collaboration with the AACN, developed gerontological nursing curriculum materials for baccalaureate nursing programs. Support from the Hartford Foundation enabled expansion of these efforts (www.hartfordign.org). Interdisciplinary educational opportunities are provided by the American Geriatrics Society and Gerontological Society of America. Federally funded GECs and the National Association of Geriatric Education Centers (www.nagec.org) provide continuing education programs about care of older adults.

Legislative, Regulatory, and Other Legal Issues

Gerontological nurses at all levels of professional practice must be knowledgeable about and comply with federal, state, and local statutes, regulations, and laws, including licensure requirements. Gerontological nurses should also be aware of how they can influence legislative and regulatory processes, identify areas in which they can become involved, and then take action when appropriate.

Gerontological nurses assume an advocate role for health promotion for older adults and recognition of the uniqueness of caring for older adults, particularly by other healthcare professionals and within other specialty organizations. Gerontological nurses influence the delivery of health care to older adults across the healthcare spectrum, such as in:

- Acute care
- Community/outpatient care facilities
- Long-term care
- Rehabilitative care
- Home health
- Public health
- Corrections facilities
- Palliative care

Gerontological nurses support evidence-based practice, which includes quality improvement and risk management activities to promote best practice with the goal of optimizing the care of older adults.

Legislative Issues

Gerontological nurses are required to be aware of statutes governing their practice at the state and federal levels and to comply with applicable statutory requirements.

They participate, whenever possible, in legislative activities that influence practice change. These goals are accomplished by: being a member of a professional organization, monitoring associations for congressional activities that have an impact on professional practice, and being a legislative advocate for the gerontological population and for gerontological nursing practice.

Regulatory Issues

Gerontological nurses must comply with state and federal regulations that govern their practice. APRNs must be knowledgeable about and follow the regulations implemented by Centers for Medicare and Medicaid, if applicable, when providing care to the gerontological population. Gerontological nurses can participate in the regulatory process by becoming a member of an expert panel or submitting formal comments to proposed regulations.

Legal Obligations and Licensure Issues

Gerontological nurses can minimize their risk of personal and professional liability by obtaining and maintaining adequate knowledge of and following federal, state, and local laws. Knowledge of laws developed and enacted for the protection of the older adult will assist gerontological nurses in guarding the health, safety, and rights of older adults and in protecting them from neglect, abuse, and exploitation.

Gerontological nurses must adhere to individual professional licensure rules and the nursing practice acts and implementing regulations governing practice in their jurisdiction and employment setting. They also must be aware of organizational policies and procedures and apply them in their daily practice. Gerontological nurses should be aware of the consequences of failing to comply with licensing rules and regulations and of failing to follow organizational policies and procedures. Consequences may include criminal charges, disciplinary action, personal and professional liability, and exclusion from governmental programs.

Gerontological nurses should be familiar and comply with patient-centered legal requirements, such as the Health Insurance Portability and Accountability Act (HIPAA). They must consider ethical issues when caring for the gerontological population. ANA's *Code of Ethics for Nurses with Interpretive Statements* and *Guide to the Code of Ethics for Nurses: Interpretation and Application* provide guidance for ethical considerations.

Other Issues in Gerontological Nursing

Planning, directing, and providing care for older adults frequently involve ethical issues, for example, reviewing an assessment of an older adult's driving ability, advanced care planning for end-of-life care, Do Not Resuscitate orders, adjudicated incompetence, and powers of attorney for healthcare purposes. Identification of transition points in the trajectory of a chronic illness and prognostication regarding the end of life are frequently difficult to make and to communicate to all stakeholders.

In 1997, the Pioneer Network initiated a movement to rebalance priorities of nursing home care now known as *culture change*. It led to models of care that incorporate flexibility and resident self-determination as the guiding or defining standard of practice. The convergence of the philosophy and goals of culture change and nursing is obvious. Thus, in 2008, an interdisciplinary panel of experts convened by a collaborative (The Hartford Institute of Geriatric Nursing New York University College of Nursing Coalition for Geriatric Nursing Organizations and the Pioneer Network) proposed recommendations for nurse competencies in nursing homes where autonomy and personal choices of residents and shared decision-making are key determinants of the care plan (Burger, Kantor, Mezey, Mitty, Kluger, Algase, et al., 2008). Symptom management (e.g., chronic pain) and supportive comfort care (e.g., end-of-life preferences) are examples of practice areas that can trigger ethical dilemmas for professional nurses.

Palliative care offers a holistic approach to the biopsychosocial, cultural, and spiritual needs of older adults throughout the trajectory of a chronic illness. "The goal of palliative care is to prevent and relieve suffering and to support the best possible quality of life for patients and their families, regardless of the stage of the disease or the need for other therapies. Palliative care is both a philosophy of care and an organized, highly structured system for delivering care. Palliative care expands traditional disease-model medical treatments to include the goals of enhancing quality of life for patient and family, optimizing function, helping with decision-making and providing opportunities for personal growth. As such, it can be delivered concurrently with life-prolonging care or as the main focus of care." (National Consensus Project for Quality Palliative Care (2009). *Clinical Practice Guidelines for Quality Palliative Care*. 2nd ed. http://www.nationalconsensusproject.org). Palliative care services are increasingly available in all care settings. Most gerontological nurses are familiar with palliative care and understand that knowing the older adult's goals of care is critical at these transition points.

Hospice care is an aspect of palliative care and, because of current Medicare regulations, focuses on the last six months of life. There is a continued need to integrate gerontological and palliative care nursing because an aging population has needs requiring the knowledge and expertise of both specialties.

The current workforce is not prepared to care for the imminent and immense influx of older adults in all settings. Although healthcare agencies know the demographic predictions, there are numerous gaps in implementing the gerontolgoical nursing competencies for RNs in hospitals (Mezey, Quinlan, Fairchild, & Vezina, 2006). There also is a lack of: a) nursing faculty educationally prepared in gerontological nursing, b) nursing faculty certified in gerontological nursing, and c) gerontological nursing preceptors and mentors for students who are the future workforce.

The wages and benefits for gerontological nurses frequently are not competitive with those of other nursing specialties. This financial disparity is especially evident in long-term care settings.

A significant amount of research in gerontological nursing has occurred over the past 20 years in the management of common conditions in older adults and settings of care (Archbold, Stewart, & Lyons, 2002). However, aging has become a public health issue requiring new approaches to care. More nurse scientists passionate about conducting research are needed to provide the evidence for interventions and healthcare policy to improve the quality and quantity of life for older adults.

All of the issues above adversely affect the recruitment and retention of qualified registered nurses interested in providing care for older adults. These issues together with the myths and stereotypic perception of aging in our society hamper recruiting highly qualified students into gerontological nursing.

These issues can be resolved if action is taken. However, if the issues remain unresolved, the cumulative impact will have significant consequences for our aging population and our overall healthcare system. Projected consequences include but are not limited to extremely high nurse-patient ratios; proliferation of high-tech, low-touch care systems; and a decline in public trust for nursing. Gerontological nurses have the expertise and passionate commitment to make the changes necessary to improve the quality of living for older adults.

Opportunities in Gerontological Nursing

The 21st century is an exciting time to be a gerontological nurse. Numerous opportunities exist for individual gerontological nurses and the gerontological nursing specialty as a whole to have a positive effect on behalf of older adults on the care, healthcare system, and environment. Participation can occur at the local level (clinical and academic settings), city, state, national, and international levels. Addressing the environment of care from the perspective of assuring the safety of older adults and their caregivers calls for the examination of working conditions and workforce issues, and the sufficient investment of human and material resources. Opportunities for action include but are not limited to:

- Developing career and leadership opportunities for gerontological nurses, such as the ANA Ethnic/Racial Clinical Fellowship Program that provides support to minority nurses during the course of their academic education;

- Incorporating gerontological educational content into nursing programs per IOM direction;

- Developing incentives to attract healthcare providers (RNs, APRNs, MDs, DOs, pharmacists, social workers, etc.) to the care of older adults;

- Continuing to develop and update evidence-based guidelines, standards of care, and effective best-practice models of care for older adults;

- Promoting healthy aging (*Healthy People 2010, Healthy People 2020*);

- Developing strategies and support for informal caregivers of older adults;

- Promoting professional certification in gerontological nursing;

- Promoting the development of nurse scientists in gerontological nursing, especially among minority nurses, by working with the five national minority nurses professional associations (Asian American Pacific Islander Nurses Association, Black Nurses Association, Hispanic/Latino Nurses Association, Native American Indian, Native Alaska Nurses Association, Philippine Nurses Association of America) and the National Coalition of Ethnic Minority Nurses Association (NCEMNA) (www.NCEMNA.org), a federally supported organization, with the goal of increasing the number of ethnic minority nurse scientists;

- Collaborating with nurse scientists in research studies;

- Using research findings related to older adults in clinical practice and teaching;

- Disseminating research findings; and

- Working diligently to increase Medicare and Medicaid reimbursement for services provided by gerontological nurses.

Healthcare providers must recognize that an older adult's presentation of acute or chronic illness is unique. The foundation of this unique presentation is the physiology of aging that also results in changes in the body's pharmacokinetics and pharmacodynamics. In addition to these normal changes of aging, the multiple chronic illnesses and conditions often experienced concurrently by the older adult can result in decreased functional ability and frailty. Older adults also experience multiple losses, which together with normal changes of aging and chronic illness may be overwhelming and result in feelings of powerlessness, loss of control, and vulnerability. Healthcare providers must also recognize the heterogeneity among older adults. All older adults are not the same. Assessment, planning, implementation, and evaluation of care must focus on the older adult as an individual and unique human being within the context of family, community, social, and cultural environments.

This scope of practice statement is meant to convey the importance of the gerontological nurse in caring for the older adult within a healthcare system confronting an unprecedented increase in the number of older adults. Adequate numbers of certified gerontological nurses, geriatricians, and other healthcare team members focused on the care of older adults must be prepared and supported with the appropriate initial education and continuing professional development programs. In addition, nurse scientists are needed to discover the evidence to support our interventions and care. The goal is to provide the highest quality of care to older adults, thereby promoting the highest quality of life.

Standards of Gerontological Nursing Practice

The standards of gerontological nursing practice are authoritative statements that identify the responsibilities for which gerontological nurses are accountable, reflect the values and priorities of gerontological nursing, are written in measurable terms, and provide a framework for the evaluation of gerontological nursing practice. The standards remain stable over time as they reflect the philosophical values of the nursing profession and specialty.

The standards are divided into two sections: the Standards of Practice and the Standards of Professional Performance. The Standards of Practice describe the application of the steps of the nursing process within practice:

- Assessment
- Diagnosis
- Outcomes identification
- Planning
- Implementation
- Evaluation

The development and maintenance of a therapeutic, holistic, nurse-older adult and family relationship are essential throughout the nursing process. The nursing process forms the foundation of clinical decision-making and encompasses all significant actions taken by the gerontological nurse in providing care for older adults, their families, and significant others. The gerontological nurse is adept at:

- Providing age-appropriate, culturally, ethnically, and spiritually sensitive physical and mental care and support;
- Adopting a lifespan perspective that appreciates the meaning and impact of ageism, poverty, and disability;
- Educating older adults and families about chronic illness and mental health care and treatment options;

- Coordinating care across settings and among caregivers, with attention to the impact of housing, diet, transportation, and importance of social networks;

- Maintaining a safe environment;

- Managing and communicating information in a prompt and efficient manner while protecting confidentiality; and

- Recognizing the importance of interprofessional collaboration in addressing the complex needs of older adults.

Function of Standards

The Standards of Gerontological Nursing Practice are authoritative statements by which nurses practicing within the role, population, and specialty governed by this document describe the duties that they are expected to competently perform. The Standards published herein may be used as evidence of the legal standard of care governing nurses practicing within the role, population, and specialty governed by this document. The Standards are subject to change with the dynamics of the nursing profession and as new patterns of professional practice are developed and accepted by the nursing profession and the public. In addition, specific conditions and clinical circumstances may also affect the application of the Standards at a given time, e.g., during a natural disaster. The Standards are subject to formal, periodic review and revision.

The measurement criteria that appear below each standard, which are not all-inclusive, do not establish the legal standard of care. Rather, these measurement criteria are specific, measurable elements that can be used by nursing professionals to measure professional performance. Nurses can identify opportunities for development and improvement by evaluating performance on these elements.

Gerontological nurses use the nursing process, the essential methodology by which older adult goals are identified and achieved. The nursing process comprises assessment, diagnosis, outcomes identification, planning, implementation, and evaluation.

Standards of Practice

Standard 1. Assessment

The gerontological nurse collects comprehensive data pertinent to the older adult's physical and mental health or situation.

Measurement Criteria

The gerontological nurse:

- Prioritizes data collection activities based on the older adult's immediate condition or needs, personal goals for physical and mental health care, cultural beliefs, socioeconomic factors, and anticipated needs;

- Collects data in a systematic and ongoing process using appropriate evidence-based, standardized assessment tools and techniques;

- Involves the older adult, family, significant others, designated caregiver, and other healthcare providers, across environments of care, as appropriate, in holistic data collection;

- Uses analytical models and problem-solving tools; and

- Documents relevant data, including risk factors and medications, in a retrievable format.

Additional Measurement Criteria for the Gerontological Advanced Practice Registered Nurse:

The gerontological advanced practice registered nurse:

- Initiates and interprets diagnostic tests and procedures relevant to the older adult current status; and

- Completes comprehensive assessments that identify the older adult's specialized needs.

STANDARD 2. DIAGNOSIS
The gerontological nurse analyzes the assessment data to determine the diagnoses or issues.

Measurement Criteria

The gerontological nurse:

- Derives the diagnoses, needs, and issues based on assessment data;

- Validates the diagnoses, needs, and issues with the older adult, family, significant others, designated caregiver, and other healthcare providers; and

- Documents diagnoses, needs, and issues in a manner that facilitates the determination of the expected outcomes and plan.

Additional Measurement Criteria for the Gerontological Advanced Practice Registered Nurse

The gerontological advanced practice registered nurse:

- Systematically compares and contrasts clinical findings with normal and abnormal variations, including co-occurring psychiatric symptoms and developmental events, in formulating a differential diagnosis;

- Uses complex data and information obtained during interview, examination, and diagnostic procedures in identifying diagnoses; and

- Assists staff in developing and maintaining competence in the diagnostic process related to the older adult.

Standard 3. Outcomes Identification
The gerontological nurse identifies expected outcomes for a plan individualized to the older adult or situation.

Measurement Criteria

The gerontological nurse:

- Involves the older adult, family, significant others, designated caregiver, and other healthcare providers in formulating expected outcomes when possible and appropriate;

- Derives culturally appropriate expected outcomes from the diagnoses;

- Considers current scientific evidence, clinical expertise, associated risks, benefits, and costs when formulating expected outcomes;

- Defines expected outcomes in terms of the older adult, older adult's values, ethical considerations, environment, and situation with consideration to current scientific evidence, associated risks, benefits, and costs;

- Includes a time estimate for attainment of expected outcomes;

- Develops expected outcomes that provide direction for continuity of care;

- Modifies expected outcomes based on changes in the status of the older adult or evaluation of the situation; and

- Documents expected outcomes as measurable goals.

Additional Measurement Criteria for the Gerontological Advanced Practice Registered Nurse:

The gerontological advanced practice registered nurse:

- Identifies expected outcomes that incorporate scientific evidence and are achievable through implementation of evidence-based practice initiatives;

- Identifies expected outcomes that incorporate clinical effectiveness and cost, older adult satisfaction, and continuity and consistency among providers; and

- Supports the use of clinical guidelines linked to positive outcomes for older adults.

STANDARD 4. PLANNING
The gerontological nurse develops a plan to attain expected outcomes.

Measurement Criteria

The gerontological nurse:

- Develops an individualized, person-centered plan considering the older adult's characteristics, personal history, and the situation;

- Develops the plan in partnership with the older adult, family, and others, as appropriate;

- Includes strategies within the plan that address each of the identified diagnoses or issues, which may include strategies for promotion and restoration of function and health; prevention of illness, injury, and disease; and end-of-life care;

- Provides for continuity within the plan, especially at all care transition points;

- Incorporates an implementation pathway or timeline within the plan;

- Establishes the plan priorities with the older adult, family, and others as appropriate;

- Uses the plan to provide direction and guidance to formal and informal caregivers and other members of the healthcare team;

- Defines the plan to reflect current statutes, rules and regulations, and standards;

- Integrates current trends and research affecting care in the planning process;

- Considers the economic impact of the plan; and

- Uses standardized language or recognized terminology to document the plan.

Additional Measurement Criteria for the Gerontological Advanced Practice Registered Nurse:

- Identifies assessment, diagnostic strategies, and therapeutic interventions within the plan that reflect current evidence, including data, research, literature and expert clinical knowledge related to care of the older adult;

- Selects or designs strategies to meet the multifaceted needs and complexity of older adults; and

- Includes the synthesis of the older adult's values and beliefs regarding nursing, medical, and complementary therapies within the plan.

STANDARD 5. IMPLEMENTATION
The gerontological nurse implements the identified plan.

Measurement Criteria

The gerontological nurse:

- Implements the plan of care in a safe and timely manner;

- Uses evidence-based interventions and treatments specific to the diagnosis or problem;

- Uses community resources and systems to implement the plan;

- Collaborates with the older adult, nursing colleagues, members of the interprofessional team, and others to implement the plan; and

- Documents implementation, any modifications, and revisions to the identified plan.

Additional Measurement Criteria for the Gerontological Advanced Practice Registered Nurse

The gerontological advanced practice registered nurse:

- Facilitates the use of systems and community resources to implement the plan;

- Supports collaboration with nursing colleagues and other disciplines to implement the plan; and

- Incorporates new knowledge and strategies to initiate change in nursing care practices to achieve optimal outcomes.

STANDARD 5A. COORDINATION OF CARE
The gerontological nurse coordinates care delivery.

Measurement Criteria:

The gerontological registered nurse:

- Coordinates implementation of the plan;

- Addresses concerns associated with transitional stages of the plan; and

- Documents the coordination of care.

Measurement Criteria for the Gerontological Advanced Practice Registered Nurse:

The gerontological advanced practice registered nurse:

- Provides leadership in the coordination of interprofessional health care for integrated delivery of care services for the older adult;

- Synthesizes data and information to prescribe necessary system and community support measures, including environmental modifications; and

- Coordinates system and community resources that enhance delivery of care across continuums.

STANDARD 5B. HEALTH TEACHING AND HEALTH PROMOTION
The gerontological registered nurse employs strategies to promote health and a safe environment.

Measurement Criteria:

The gerontological registered nurse:

- Provides health teaching that addresses such topics as healthy lifestyles, risk-reducing behaviors, developmental needs, activities of daily living, and preventive self-care;

- Uses health promotion and health teaching methods appropriate to the situation and the older adult's developmental level, learning needs, cognitive status, readiness and ability to learn, language preference, and culture; and

- Seeks opportunities for feedback and evaluation of the effectiveness of the strategies used.

Additional Measurement Criteria for the Gerontological Advanced Practice Registered Nurse:

The gerontological advanced practice registered nurse:

- Synthesizes empirical evidence on risk behaviors, learning theories, behavioral change theories, motivational theories, epidemiology, and other related theories and frameworks when designing health information and education for the older adult;

- Designs health information and education programs and materials appropriate to the older adult's developmental level, learning needs, readiness and ability to learn, and cultural values and beliefs; and

- Evaluates health information resources, such as the Internet, within the area of practice for accuracy, readability, and comprehensibility to help older adults access quality health information.

STANDARD 5C. CONSULTATION

The gerontological advanced practice registered nurse provides consultation to influence the identified plan, enhance the abilities of others, and effect change.

Measurement Criteria for the Gerontological Advanced Practice Registered Nurse:

The gerontological advanced practice registered nurse:

- Synthesizes clinical data, theoretical frameworks, and evidence when providing consultation;

- Facilitates the effectiveness of a consultation by involving the older adult in decision-making and negotiating role responsibilities and, as necessary, family and significant others; and

- Communicates consultation recommendations that facilitate change.

STANDARD 5D. PRESCRIPTIVE AUTHORITY AND TREATMENT
The gerontological advanced practice registered nurse uses prescriptive authority, procedures, referrals, treatments, and therapies in accordance with state and federal laws and regulations.

Measurement Criteria for the Gerontological Advanced Practice Registered Nurse:

The gerontological advanced practice registered nurse:

- Prescribes evidence-based treatments, therapies, and procedures considering the older adult's comprehensive healthcare needs;

- Prescribes pharmacologic agents based on current evidence of age-related pharmacokinetic and pharmacodynamic changes, pharmacology, and pathophysiology;

- Prescribes specific pharmacological and nonpharmacological agents and/or treatments based on clinical indicators, the older adult's status and needs, and the results of diagnostic and laboratory tests;

- Evaluates therapeutic and potential adverse effects, including psychiatric and cognitive symptoms, of pharmacological and non-pharmacological treatments;

- Provides older adults and their caregivers with information about intended effects and potential adverse effects of proposed prescriptive therapies; and

- Provides information about costs, treatment options, and their risks and benefits as appropriate.

STANDARD 6. EVALUATION
The gerontological registered nurse evaluates progress toward attainment of outcomes.

Measurement Criteria:

The gerontological nurse:

- Conducts a systematic, ongoing, and criterion-based evaluation of the outcomes in relation to the structures and processes prescribed by the plan and the indicated timeline;

- Partners with the older adult and others involved in the care or situation in the evaluative process;

- Evaluates the effectiveness of the planned strategies in relation to the older adult's responses and the attainment of the expected outcomes;

- Documents the results of the evaluation;

- Uses ongoing assessment data to revise the diagnoses, outcomes, plan, and implementation as needed; and

- Disseminates the results to the older adult and others involved in the care or situation, as appropriate, in accordance with state and federal laws and regulations.

Additional Measurement Criteria for the Gerontological Advanced Practice Registered Nurse:

The geronotological advanced practice registered nurse:

- Evaluates the accuracy of the diagnosis and effectiveness of the interventions in relationship to the older adult's attainment of expected outcomes;

- Synthesizes the results of the evaluation to determine the impact of the plan on the older adult, family, groups, communities, organizations, and institutions; and

- Uses the results of the evaluation to make or recommend process or structural changes, including policy, procedure, and protocol documentation, as appropriate.

STANDARDS OF PROFESSIONAL PERFORMANCE

STANDARD 7. QUALITY OF PRACTICE
The gerontological registered nurse systematically enhances the quality and effectiveness of nursing practice.

Measurement Criteria:

The gerontological registered nurse:

- Demonstrates quality by documenting the application of the nursing process in a responsible, accountable, and ethical manner;

- Uses the results of quality improvement activities to initiate changes in nursing practice and in the healthcare delivery system;

- Incorporates new knowledge to initiate changes in nursing practice if desired outcomes are not achieved;

- Evaluates quality of service provided in conjunction with older adults and their families;

- Obtains and maintains professional certification in gerontological nursing and other certifications as appropriate; and

- Participates in quality improvement activities.

Additional Measurement Criteria for the Gerontological Advanced Practice Registered Nurse:

The gerontological advanced practice registered nurse:

- Obtains and maintains gerontological nursing advanced practice certification;

- Designs quality improvement initiatives;

- Implements initiatives to evaluate the need for change;

- Evaluates the practice environment and quality of nursing care rendered in relation to existing evidence, identifying opportunities for the generation and use of research; and

- Implements processes to remove or decrease barriers within organizational systems.

STANDARD 8. PROFESSIONAL PRACTICE EVALUATION

The gerontological registered nurse evaluates his or her own nursing practice in relation to professional practice standards and guidelines and relevant statutes, rules, and regulations.

Measurement Criteria:

The gerontological registered nurse:

- Provides care in a culturally and ethnically sensitive manner;

- Engages in self-evaluation of practice on a regular basis, identifying areas of strength as well as areas in which professional development would be beneficial;

- Obtains informal feedback regarding the practice from older adults, peers, professional colleagues, and others;

- Participates in systematic peer review as appropriate;

- Takes action to achieve goals identified during the evaluation process;

- Provides rationales for practice beliefs, decisions, and actions as part of the informal and formal evaluation processes; and

- Provides feedback to other nurses as appropriate to improve gerontological nursing practice.

Additional Measurement Criteria for the Gerontological Advanced Practice Registered Nurse:

The gerontological advanced practice registered nurse: Engages in a formal process, seeking feedback regarding his or her own practice from patients, peers, professional colleagues, and others.

STANDARD 9. EDUCATION
The gerontological registered nurse attains knowledge and competence that reflects current gerontological nursing practice.

Measurement Criteria:

The gerontological registered nurse:

- Identifies personal gerontological educational needs through ongoing self-reflection and inquiry;

- Participates in gerontological education based on individual learning needs and practice setting;

- Demonstrates a commitment to lifelong learning to keep current with evidence-based practice and the changing health and social needs of the older adult;

- Seeks experiences that reflect current practice in order to maintain skills and competence in clinical practice and role performance;

- Acquires knowledge and skills appropriate to the specialty area, practice setting, role, and situation;

- Maintains current interpersonal, technical, and information technology competencies that are consistent with nursing practice in the care of older adults;

- Shares best practices by participating in nursing and interprofessional educational programs, conferences, workshops, and meetings;

- Maintains professional records that provide evidence of competence and lifelong learning; and

- Serves as a role model to nursing students, nursing team members, and others.

Additional Measurement Criteria for the Gerontological Advanced Practice Registered Nurse:

The gerontological advanced practice registered nurse:

- Uses current healthcare research findings and other evidence to expand clinical knowledge, enhance role performance, and increase knowledge of gerontological and other professional issues;

Continued ▶

- Provides in-service, continuing, and community education in gerontology to others;

- Presents and or publishes on content expertise in gerontology;

- Serves as a resource to other advanced practice nurses in the area of gerontology; and

- Mentors or precepts nursing and other professional students.

STANDARD 10. COLLEGIALITY
The gerontological registered nurse interacts with and contributes to the professional development of peers and colleagues.

Measurement Criteria:

The gerontological registered nurse:

- Shares knowledge and skills with peers and colleagues in nursing and across disciplines by such activities as older adult care conferences, presentations at formal or informal meetings, journal clubs, and online lists;

- Provides peers and colleagues with feedback regarding their practice and role performance;

- Interacts with peers and colleagues to enhance professional nursing practice and role performance;

- Maintains supportive relationships with peers and colleagues that increase the effectiveness of a team, unit, or agency;

- Contributes to an environment that is conducive to the education of healthcare professionals; and

- Contributes to a supportive and healthy workplace.

Additional Measurement Criteria for the Gerontological Advanced Practice Registered Nurse:

The gerontological advanced practice registered nurse:

- Models expert practice to interprofessional team members and consumers; and

- Participates in interprofessional teams that contribute to role development, advanced-level gerontological nursing practice, and research.

STANDARD 11. COLLABORATION

The gerontological registered nurse collaborates with the older adult, family and significant others, interprofessional team, community, and other stakeholders in the conduct of nursing practice.

Measurement Criteria:

The gerontological registered nurse:

- Communicates with the older adult, the family, significant others, designated caregivers, interprofessional team and healthcare providers, community, and other stakeholders regarding care of the older adult and the nurse's role in the provision of that care;

- Collaborates in creating a documented plan, focused on outcomes and decisions related to care and delivery of services, that indicates communication with older adults, families, significant others, the interdisciplinary team, and relevant others;

- Partners with others to effect change and generate positive outcomes through knowledge of the older adult, family, significant others, and situation; and

- Documents referrals, including provisions for continuity of care.

Additional Measurement Criteria for the Gerontological Advanced Practice Registered Nurse:

The gerontological advanced practice registered nurse:

- Partners with other professionals to enhance older adult care through interprofessional activities such as education, consultation, management, technological development, and research opportunities;

- Facilitates an interprofessional process with other members of the healthcare team and community; and

- Documents plan-of-care communications, rationales for plan-of-care changes, and collaborative discussions to improve care of the older adult.

STANDARD 12. ETHICS
The gerontological nurse integrates ethical provisions in all areas of practice.

Measurement Criteria:

The gerontological registered nurse:

- Uses *Code of Ethics for Nurses with Interpretive Statements* (ANA, 2001) to guide practice;

- Delivers care in a manner that preserves and protects autonomy, cultural preferences, dignity, and rights and honors the wishes of the older adult;

- Maintains confidentiality of information about care of the older adult within legal and regulatory parameters;

- Actively participates in the informed consent process (including the right to choose) for the older adult's procedures, tests, treatments, and research participation, as appropriate, by educating, advocating, and clarifying options to the older adult, family, and significant others;

- Serves as an advocate in assisting older adults in developing skills for self-advocacy;

- Serves as an advocate reporting suspected abuse and neglect of the older adult;

- Maintains a therapeutic and professional older adult-nurse relationship within appropriate professional boundaries;

- Contributes to resolving ethical issues of older adults, colleagues, and systems as evidenced in such activities as requesting an ethics consult in a confidential, nonpunitive manner;

- Reports illegal, incompetent, and impaired practices; and

- Demonstrates a commitment to practicing self-care, managing stress, and connecting with self and others.

Continued ▶

Additional Measurement Criteria for the Gerontological Advanced Practice Registered Nurse:

The gerontological advanced practice registered nurse:

- Informs the older adult of the risks, benefits, and outcomes of healthcare regimens; and

- Participates in interprofessional teams that address ethical risks, benefits, and outcomes of practice.

STANDARD 13. RESEARCH
The gerontological nurse integrates research findings into practice.

Measurement Criteria:

The gerontological registered nurse:

- Utilizes the best available evidence, including research findings, to guide practice decisions;

- Actively participates in research activities at various levels appropriate to the nurse's level of education and position, such as:

  - Identifying clinical problems suitable for gerontological nursing research (care of older adults and nursing practice;

  - Participating in data collection (surveys, pilot projects, and formal studies;

  - Participating in a formal committee or program;

  - Sharing research activities and findings with peers and others;

  - Participating in research studies;

  - Using research findings in the development of policies, procedures, and standards of practice for care of older adults;

  - Incorporating research as a basis for learning; and

- Advocates for the rights and welfare of individuals who participate as subjects in research activities

Additional Measurement Criteria for the Gerontological Advanced Practice Registered Nurse:

The gerontological advanced practice registered nurse:

- Contributes to nursing knowledge by conducting or synthesizing research that discovers, examines, and evaluates knowledge, theories, criteria, and creative approaches to improve healthcare practices in the care of older adults;

- Formally disseminates research findings through activities such as presentations, publications, consultations, listservs, and journal clubs;

Continued ▶

- Conducts analyses that interpret research for application to practice; and

- Develops evidence-based education programs to improve and standardize the delivery of evidence-based care for the interdisciplinary team.

STANDARD 14. RESOURCE UTILIZATION
The gerontological nurse considers factors related to safety, effectiveness, cost, and impact on practice in planning and delivering nursing services.

Measurement Criteria:

The gerontological registered nurse:

- Evaluates factors such as safety, effectiveness, availability, costs and benefits, efficiencies, and impact on practice when choosing practice options for the older adult that would result in the same expected outcome;

- Assists the older adult and family in identifying and securing appropriate and available services to address health-related issues and needs of the older adult;

- Assigns or delegates tasks based on the needs and condition of the older adult, potential for harm, stability of the older adult's condition, complexity of the task, and predictability of the outcome;

- Assists the older adult, family, and significant others in becoming informed consumers about the options, costs, risks, and benefits of treatment and care of the older adult, as well as state and federal regulations and the implications of those regulations related to the delivery of care; and

- Uses organizational and community resources to formulate interprofessional plans of care.

Additional Measurement Criteria for the Gerontological Advanced Practice Registered Nurse:

The gerontological advanced practice registered nurse:

- Coordinates policies, programs, and organizational and community resource efforts to meet the needs of older adults and their families;

- Develops innovative solutions for problems related to the care of the older adult that address effective resource utilization, maintenance of quality, and the older adult's goals; and

- Develops evaluation strategies to demonstrate safety, quality, cost-effectiveness, costs and benefits, and efficiency factors associated with nursing practice.

STANDARD 15. LEADERSHIP

The gerontological registered nurse provides leadership in the professional practice setting and the profession.

Measurement criteria:

The gerontological registered nurse:

- Engages in teamwork as a team player, a team builder, and team leader;

- Works to create and maintain healthy work environments in local, regional, national, and international communities;

- Demonstrates the ability to create a shared vision, the associated goals, and a plan to implement and measure progress;

- Demonstrates a commitment to continuous, lifelong learning for self and others;

- Facilitates teaching others to succeed by mentoring and other strategies;

- Exhibits creativity and flexibility through times of change;

- Demonstrates energy, excitement, and a passion for quality work;

- Willingly acknowledges mistakes by self and others, thereby creating a culture in which risk-taking is not only safe, but expected;

- Inspires loyalty by valuing of people as the most precious asset in an organization;

- Directs the coordination of care across settings and among caregivers, including oversight of licensed and unlicensed personnel in any assigned or delegated tasks;

- Serves in key roles in the work setting by participating on committees, councils, and administrative teams; and

- Promotes advancement of the profession through participation in professional organizations.

Additional Measurement Criteria for the Gerontological Advanced Practice Registered Nurse:

The gerontological advanced practice registered nurse:

- Works to influence local, state, regional, national, and international decision-making bodies to improve care of the older adult;

- Provides direction to enhance the effectiveness of the healthcare team;

- Initiates and revises protocols or guidelines to reflect evidence-based practice, to reflect accepted changes in care management, and to address emerging problems;

- Promotes communication of information and advancement of the profession through writing, publishing, and presentation for professional and lay audiences; and

- Designs innovation to effect change in practice and improve health outcomes.

STANDARD 16. ADVOCACY
The gerontological nurse advocates to protect the health, safety, and rights of the older adult.

Measurement Criteria:

The gerontological registered nurse:

- Empowers older adults and families in health literacy for decision-making and healthcare management;

- Respects the moral and legal rights of individuals, families, community, groups, and populations;

- Intercedes on behalf of older adults and families who have difficulty navigating the healthcare system;

- Facilitates person-centered care, which includes actions such as "identify, respect, and care about older adult differences, values, preferences, and expressed needs" (IOM, 2003);

- Ensures dignified and humane care of older adults and their families;

- Safeguards the older adult's and family's rights to privacy and confidentiality;

- Identifies the nurse's role as a member of an interprofessional team in providing high-quality care and safety of the older adult;

- Monitors healthcare resources to promote equitable care of older adults;

- Identifies generational differences in the workforce and workplace; and

- Advocates for gerontological issues in work organization and political settings.

Additional Measurement Criteria for the Gerontological Advanced Practice Registered Nurse:

The gerontological advanced practice registered nurse:

- Educates about advocacy for individuals, families, community, groups, and populations; and

- Leads advocacy actions related to the care of older adults, especially those with complex health issues.

GLOSSARY

Advanced practice gerontological nurse. A nurse practitioner and/or clinical specialist who holds at least a master's degree in nursing, has advanced clinical experience, and demonstrates extensive knowledge, competence, and skill in the care of older adults as validated by a national certifying organization.

Assessment. A systematic, dynamic process by which the registered nurse, through interaction with the patient, family, groups, communities, populations, and healthcare providers, collects and analyzes data. This may include physical, psychological, socio-cultural, spiritual, cognitive, functional abilities, developmental, economic, and lifestyle dimensions.

Assisted living. A residential or facility-based program that provides, in return for payment, services and care for residents who are unable to perform or need assistance in performing the instrumental activities of daily living. Such care is provided in a way that promotes optimum dignity and independence.

Caregiver. A person who provides direct care for older adults, whether paid to do so (formal) or voluntary (informal)l such as a family member.

Certification. The formal process by which clinical competence is validated by a certifying organization in the specialty area of practice.

Code of Ethics for Nurses. The set of provisions that makes explicit the primary ethical duties, goals, values, and obligations of the nursing profession and so shape nursing practice. (ANA, 2001).

Collaboration. An interactive process whereby nurses and other healthcare professionals and caregivers work together for the benefit of the older adult in a manner that demonstrates a shared philosophy of care and mutual respect.

Competency. An expected level of performance that integrates knowledge, skills, abilities, and judgment (ANA, 2008, p. 3).

Continuity of care. An interdisciplinary process that: includes patients, families, and significant others in the development of a coordinated plan of care; and facilitates the patient's transition between settings and healthcare providers, based on changing needs and available resources.

Criteria. *See* Measurement criteria

Data. Discrete entities that are described objectively without interpretation.

Diagnosis. A clinical judgment about the patient's response to actual or potential health conditions or needs. The diagnosis provides the basis for determination of a plan to achieve expected outcomes. Registered nurses utilize nursing and/or medical diagnoses depending upon educational and clinical preparation and legal authority.

Environment. The atmosphere, milieu, or conditions in which an individual lives, works or plays.

Evaluation. The process of determining the progress toward attainment of expected outcomes, including the effectiveness of care, when addressing one's practice.

Expected outcomes. End results that are measurable, desirable, and observable, and translate into observable behaviors.

Evidence-based practice. A process founded on the collection, interpretation, and integration of valid, important, and applicable patient-reported, clinician-observed, and research-derived evidence. The best available evidence, moderated by patient circumstances and preferences, is applied to improve the quality of clinical judgments.

Family. Family of origin or significant others as identified by the patient.

Gerontological nurse. The healthcare professional who is consistently responsible for the 24-hour care of older adults across clinical settings by providing direct care and coordinating services as well as by advocacy, consultation, education, management, and research activities related to aging and its effect on older adults.

Gerontological nursing. An evidence-based nursing practice specialty that addresses the unique physiological, psychosocial, developmental, economic, cultural, and spiritual needs related to the process of aging and care of older adults. Gerontological nurses collaborate with older adults and their significant others to promote autonomy, wellness, optimal functioning, comfort, and quality of life from healthy aging to end of life. Gerontological nurses lead interprofessional teams in a holistic, person-centered approach in the specialized care of older adults.

Gerontology. The scientific study of all aspects of the aging process, including physical, psychosocial, spiritual, economic, and disease related.

Geropsychiatric nursing. The subspecialty of psychiatric nursing that addresses the mental health of older adults in an integral, interdisciplinary manner.

Guidelines. Systematically developed statements that describe recommended actions based on available scientific evidence and expert opinion. Clinical guidelines describe a process of patient care management that has the potential of improving the quality of clinical and consumer decision-making.

Health. An experience that is often expressed in terms of wellness and illness, and may occur in the presence or absence of disease or injury.

Healthcare provider. An individual with special expertise who provide healthcare services or assistance to patients, including nurses, physicians, psychologists, social workers, nutritionists, dietitians, and various therapists.

Holistic. Based on an understanding that the parts of a patient are intimately interconnected and that physical, mental, social, and spiritual factors need to be included in any interventions. The whole is a system that is greater than the sum of its parts.

Illness. The subjective experience of discomfort.

Implementation. Activities such as teaching, monitoring, providing, counseling, delegating, and coordinating.

Information. Data that are interpreted, organized, or structured.

Interdisciplinary. Reliant on the overlapping skills and knowledge of each team member and discipline, resulting in synergistic effects where outcomes are enhanced and more comprehensive than the simple aggregation of any team member's individual efforts.

Measurement criteria. Relevant, measurable indicators of the standards of practice and professional performance.

Patient. Recipient of nursing practice, used to provide consistency and brevity, understanding that the term *client, individual, resident, family, groups, communities,* or *populations* might be a more appropriate choice.

Peer review. A collegial, systematic, and periodic process by which registered nurses are held accountable for practice and which fosters the refinement of one's knowledge, skills, and decision-making at all levels and in all areas of practice.

Plan. A comprehensive outline of the components that need to be addressed to attain expected outcomes.

Rehabilitation. An interdisciplinary process that focuses on returning the older adult to their highest possible level of psychological and physical health and functional ability.

Restorative care. A philosophy of care that focuses on regaining and maintaining the highest possible functional level of the older adult.

Quality of care. The degree to which health services for patients, families, groups, communities, or populations increase the likelihood of desired outcomes and are consistent with current professional knowledge.

Scope of gerontological nursing practice. A range of gerontological nursing functions that are differentiated according to the level of practice, the role of the nurse, and the work setting. The parameters are determined by each state's nurse practice act, the Code of Ethics for Nurses, and the standards of gerontological nursing practice in this publication, along with each individual's personal competency to perform particular activities or functions.

Situation. A set of circumstances, conditions, or events.

Standard. An authoritative statement defined and promoted by a given profession by which the quality of professional practice, service, or education can be evaluated.

Standards of gerontological nursing practice. Authoritative statements that identify the responsibilities for which gerontological nurses are accountable, reflect the values and priorities of gerontological nursing, are written in measurable terms, and provide a framework for the evaluation of gerontological nursing practice.

Strategy. A plan of action to achieve a major overall goal.

Theory (nursing). A set of interrelated concepts, definitions, or propositions used to systematically describe, explain, predict, or control human responses or phenomena of interest to nurses. (ANA 2010; pg. 42)

REFERENCES

All URLs were retrieved on August 30, 2010.

American Nurses Association. (2001a). *Scope and standards of geronto-logical nursing practice, second edition.* Silver Spring, MD: Nursesbooks.org.

American Nurses Association. (2001b). *Code of ethics for nurses with interpretive statements.* Silver Spring, MD: Nursesbooks.org.

American Nurses Association. (2004). *Nursing: Scope and standards of practice.* Silver Spring, MD: Nursesbooks.org.

American Nurses Association (ANA). (2008). *Position statement: Professional role competence.* Silver Spring, MD: Author. http://www.nursingworld.org/NursingPractice

American Nurses Association (ANA). (2010). *Nursing's social policy statement: The essencs of the profession.* Silver Spring, MD: Nursesbooks.org.

Brush, B.L. (2008). Global nurse migration today. *Journal of Nursing Scholarship,* 40(1), 20–25.

Burnside, I. M. (1981). *Nursing the aged, second edition.* New York: McGraw Hill, Inc.

Burger, S.G., Kantor, B., Mezey, M., Mitty, E., Kluger, M., Algase, D., Anderson, K., Beck, C., Mueller, C., & Rader, J. (2009). *Issue Paper: Nurses' involvement in nursing home culture change: Overcoming barriers, advancing opportunities.* (Spring.) The Hartford Institute of Geriatric Nursing, New York University College of Nursing, Coalition for Geriatric Nursing Organizations, and The Pioneer Network. New York: Hartford Institute. http://hartfordign.org/policy/position_papers_briefs

Capzuti, E., Zwicker, D., Mezey, M., Fulmer, T. (Eds). (2008) *Evidence-based geriatric nursing protocols for best practice, third edition.* New York: Springer Publishing Company.

Crystal, S., Sambamoorghi, U.,Walkup, J. T., & Akincigial, A. (2003). Diagnosis and treatment of depression in the elderly Medicare population: Predictors, disparities, and trends. *Journal of the American Geriatrics Society, 51*, 1718-1728.

Eliopoulos, C. (2010). Preface, in: *Gerontological nursing, seventh edition*. Philadelphia: Lippincott, Williams & Wilkins.

Fowler, M. D. M. (Ed.). (2008). *Guide to the code of ethics for nurses: Interpretation and application*. Silver Spring, MD: Nursesbooks.org.

Hartford Institute for Geriatric Nursing. (2010). *Professional nursing associations creating and/or revising professional scope and standards: Guidelines for addressing issues related to care of older adults*. New York: Author. http://consultgerirn.org/uploads/File/scopes_standards.pdf

Hoover, D. R., Crystal, S., Kumar, R., Sambamoorthi, U. & Cantor, J. C. (2002). Medical expenditures during the last year of life: Findings from the 1992–1996 Medicare current beneficiary survey. *Health Services Research, 37*(6), 1625–1642.

Institute of Medicine. (2003). *Health professions education: Bridge to quality*. Washington, DC: National Academies Press.

Institute of Medicine. (2008). *Retooling for an aging America: Building the health care workforce*. Washington, DC: National Academies Press.

Kelly, T.B., Tolson, D., Schofield, I., & Booth, J. (2005). Describing gerontological nursing: An academic exercise or prerequisite for progress. *International Journal of Nursing Older People 14* (3a), 1–11

Mezey, M., Stierle, L.J., Huba, G.J., & Esterson, J. (2007) Ensuring competence of specialty nurses in care of older adults. *Geriatric Nursing 28*(6S):9–14. (Special Issue, November/December.)

National Consensus Project for Quality Palliative Care (2009). *Clinical practice guidelines for quality palliative care, second edition*. Washington, DC: Author. http://www.nationalconsensusproject.org.

National League for Nursing (2008). *Preparing the next generation of nurses to practice in a technology-rich environment: An informatics agenda.* Chicago: Author. http://www.nln.org/aboutnln/PositionStatements/informatics_052808.pdf

Stierle, L. J., Mezey, M., Schumann, M. J., Esterson, J., Smolenski, M. C., Horsley, K. D., Rotunda, N., Brenner, B. R., Paulson, D., Huba, G. J., & Gould, E. (2006). The nurse competence in aging initiative: Encouraging expertise in the care of older adults. *American Journal of Nursing, 106*(9), 93–96.

ADDITIONAL RESOURCES

All URLs were retrieved on August 30, 2010.

American Association of Colleges of Nursing & The John A. Hartford Foundation Institute for Geriatric Nursing (2006). *Caring for an aging America: A guide for faculty.* http://www.aacn.nche.edu/Education/ Hartford/pdf/monograph.pdf

American Association of Colleges of Nursing & The John A. Hartford Foundation Institute for Geriatric Nursing (2000*). Older adults: Curriculum guidelines for geriatric nursing care.* Retrieved http://www.aacn .nche.edu/Education/gercomp.htm

American Nurses Association (2008). *Home health nursing: Scope and standards of practice.* Silver Spring, MD: Nursesbooks.org.

Annual Review of Nursing Research: Geriatric nursing research. Volume 20, 2002. Joyce J. Fitzpatrick, Series Editor; Patricia G. Archbold and Barbara J. Stewart, Volume Editors; Karen S. Lyons, Associate Editor.

APRN Joint Dialogue Group (2008). *Consensus Model for APRN Regulation: Licensure, accreditation, certification and education.* http://www .nursingworld.org/DocumentVault/APRN-Resource-Section/APRN-Consensus-Model-FAQ.aspx

Butcher, H. K. (2006). Re-envisioning gerontological mental health nursing education.

Journal of the American Psychiatric Nurses Association 12(2), 116–120.

Ebersole, P., Hess, P., Touhy, T., & Jett., K. (2005). *Gerontological nursing and healthy aging.* St. Louise: Mosby Elsevier.

Ebersole, P. & Touhy, T. (2006). *Geriatric nursing: Growth of a specialty.* New York: Springer.

National Consensus Project for Quality Palliative Care. (2009) *Clinical practice guidelines for quality palliative care, second edition*.www .nationalconsensusproject.org

Hartford Geriatric Nursing Initiative (2004). *Nurse Practitioner and the Clinical Nurse Specialist competencies for the older adult care*. New York: Author. http://www.aacn.nche.edu/Education/pdf,APNCompetencies .pdf

Hartford Institute for Geriatric Nursing. Scopes and Standards. ANA Scope & Standards of Practice: Enhancing the Care to Older Adults. http:// consultgerirn.org/resources/Scopes_and_Standards/ANA

Kolanowski, A., & Piven, M. (2006). Geropsychiatric nursing: The state of the science. *Journal of the American psychiatric nurses association*. 12(2), 75–99.

Luggen, A.S., & Meiner, S.E. (2001). *NGNA: Core curriculum for geronto- logical nursing, second edition*. St. Louis: Mosby.

Meiner, S.E., & Lueckenotte, A.G. (2006). *Gerontologic nursing, third edition*. St. Louis, MO: Mosby Elsevier.

Mezey, M., Quinlan, E., Fairchild, & Vezina, M. (2006). Geriatric compe- tencies for RNs in hospitals. *Journal for Nursing in Staff Development, 22*(1), 2–10.

Morris, D., & Mentes, J. (2006). Geropsychiatric nursing education: Chal- lenge and opportunity. *Journal of the American psychiatric nurses association*. 12(2), 105–115.

National Association of Clinical Nurse Specialists (2007). *A vision of the future for Clinical Nurse Specialists*. Philadelphia: Author.

Puentes, W. J., Buckwalter, K., & Evans, L. K. (2006). Geropsychiatric nurs- ing: planning for the future. *Journal of American Psychiatric Nurses Association*. (12)2, 165–169.

APPENDIX A.
SCOPE AND STANDARDS OF GERONTOLOGICAL NURSING, SECOND EDITION (2001)

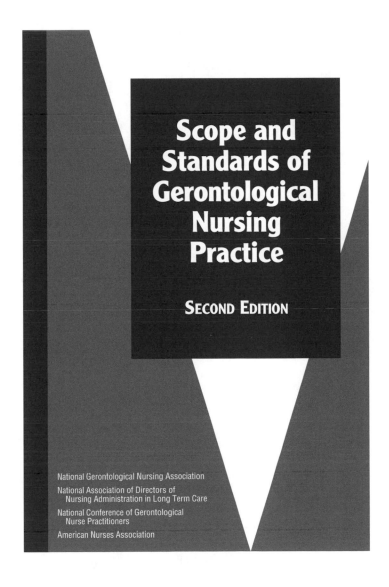

Scope and
Standards of
Gerontological
Nursing
Practice

SECOND EDITION

National Gerontological Nursing Association

National Association of Directors of
Nursing Administration in Long Term Care

National Conference of Gerontological
Nurse Practitioners

American Nurses Association

Library of Congress Cataloging-in-Publication Data

Scope and standards of gerontological nursing practice; chairperson, JoAnn G. Congdon . . . [et al.]. — 2nd ed. / National Gerontological Nursing Association, National Association of Directors of Nursing Administration in Long Term Care, National Conference of Gerontological Nurse Practitioners, American Nurses Association
    p. cm.
Includes bibliographical references.
    ISBN 1-55810-159-4
    I. Congdon, JoAnn G. II. American Nurses Association. III. American Nurses Association. Council on Gerontological Nursing. Executive Committee. Scope and standards of gerontological nursing practice.
    RC954 .A46 2001
    610.73'65'021873—dc21

                                                          2001046412

Published by
Nursesbooks.org
The Publishing Program of ANA

American Nurses Association
8515 Georgia Avenue, Suite 400
Silver Spring, MD 20910–3492

ISBN-13: 978-1-55810-159-3   ISBN-10: 1-55810-159-4

ACKNOWLEDGMENTS

The American Nurses Association gratefully acknowledges all the valuable assistance, comments, and recommendations given by various individuals and groups across the country who have collaborated throughout this revision process.

Workgroup to Review and Revise the *Scope and Standards of Gerontological Nursing Practice*

JoAnn G. Congdon, PhD, RN, CNS, Chairperson
National Gerontological Nursing Association

Jean DeCamp, RN, C, FACDONA
National Association of Directors of Nursing Administration
  in Long Term Care

Kathleen Fletcher, MSN, RN, CS, GNP
National Conference of Gerontological Nurse Practitioners

Bonnie Henningson, MPH, RN, C
National Gerontological Nursing Association

Kathleen Kaplan, RN, C
National Gerontological Nursing Association

Barbara Resnick, PhD, CRNP
University of Maryland, Baltimore, School of Nursing
  American Academy of Nurse Practitioners

Congress of Nursing Practice and Economics Liaisons

Judith Sweeney, MS, RN, CS

Sylvia Weber, MS, RN, CS

Staff, ANA Department of Nursing Practice

Carol J. Bickford, PhD, RN, BC, Senior Policy Fellow

Winifred Carson, JD, Nursing Practice Counsel

Yvonne Humes, BBA, Senior Administrative Assistant

CONTENTS

INTRODUCTION

Background

The American Nurses Association (ANA) is responsible for defining the scope and standards of nursing practice. In fulfillment of that responsibility, the first combined document of *Scope and Standards of Gerontological Nursing* was published by the ANA in 1987. This fourth revision builds on the previously established scope statement and standards of gerontological nursing practice (ANA 1976, 1981,1987, 1995). The preparation of this document included an extensive field review process, and reflects a collaboration between the ANA and several national nursing associations and organizations. It provides nursing with a common language and consistent format to articulate the scope and standards of gerontological nursing practice.

Scope and Standards of Gerontological Nursing Practice, 2nd Edition is intended to be used as a guide to current practice and in conjunction with other documents that articulate the values of professional nursing. Given the dynamic nature of healthcare in general, and of nursing specifically, this document represents the scope and practice of gerontological nursing in today's society. As with other specialty practice areas, the scope and standards for gerontological nursing practice will continue to evolve as research, public policy, consumers, and expectations change.

Application

The *Scope and Standards of Gerontological Nursing Practice, 2nd Edition* applies to gerontological nursing in clinical practice across all settings, from institutions and ambulatory care centers to alternative living and home care in the community. This publication includes the scope of gerontological nursing practice and the standards of care and standards of professional performance of gerontological nursing practice. While the *Standards of Clinical Nursing Practice, 2nd Edition* (ANA 1998) apply to all professional nurses, the gerontological standards contain specific criteria for defining expectations and competent care associated with the basic and advanced clinical practice of gerontological nursing.

Just as the nursing profession responds to the ever-changing needs and demands of healthcare, these standards and description of scope of practice will require ongoing refinement as our gerontological nursing practice evolves. We have a continual challenge to meet the changing healthcare needs of older adults in America.

SCOPE OF
PRACTICE FOR GERONTOLOGICAL NURSING

As early as the 1920s, a few visionary nurses called for the development of gerontological nursing practice. They recognized that, within the full scope of nursing practice, a body of knowledge and skills related to nursing care for older adults across all settings was uniquely distinguishable.

Gerontological nursing practice continues to evolve in our current dynamic healthcare environment with its increasing focus on aging issues related to quality of care, quality of life, access to and affordability of healthcare, ethics, and the right to detailed advance directives. In this constantly changing environment, it is helpful to delineate current assumptions, myths, characteristics of aging, tenets of gerontological nursing, and trends in population and services. The scope of practice is further differentiated between basic and advanced gerontological nursing practice.

Assumptions of Aging

The practice of gerontological nursing involves various assumptions of aging that drive the approach and philosophy of care. These include:

- Aging is a progressive, irreversible, and natural process that begins at conception.

- Older adults can age with high mental and physical function.

- The percentage of older Americans will continue to increase as life expectancy in the United States increases.

- Aging encompasses physical, emotional, psychological, sociological, and spiritual changes.

- Older adults are a heterogeneous population with varied cultural beliefs and life experiences that contribute to individual well-being and quality of life.

- Older adults seek self-fulfillment and interaction with their environment.

- Older adults are capable and desire to make informed decisions on how they live and how they die.

- Older adults often experience multiple, interacting, acute, and chronic conditions.

- The older adult's atypical response to many diseases and illnesses often delays prompt diagnosis and treatment.

Myths of Aging

Myths of aging have a negative impact because they can decrease the older adult's sense of self-confidence and can increase dependence. Society's acceptance of various myths of aging negatively affects the quality of healthcare and quality of life for older Americans. Common myths include and are not limited to the following:

- Aging is synonymous with disease and frailty.

- Older adults are unable to learn new skills.

- Older adults are rigid and resist change.

- Older adults eventually become cognitively impaired.

- Older adults are unproductive and no longer contribute to society.

- Older adults are sexless.

- Depression is normal for older adults.

- Aging is only genetically determined.

- Most older adults experience incontinence.

(Portions of content adapted from Rowe and Kahn 1998)

Common Characteristics of Aging

Although older adults respond individually to the aging process, they also share many common characteristics of aging. Examples include:

- Physical changes occur at various rates in older adults. Tissue and cell changes affect the immune response and the ability to respond to various hormones and sensory input.

- Social interaction, individual coping skills, life experiences and losses, as well as role perception, spiritual, and cultural beliefs all affect aging.

- Older adults can take the necessary precautions to minimize risks to their well-being if they know the physiologic changes caused by physical, emotional, mental, or spiritual stress. Examples of these changes may include a decreased sense of thirst, prolonged time for visual accommodation, and decreased ability to thermoregulate body temperature to adjust to the environment.

- Exercise benefits older adults by increasing physical and mental health and well-being.

- Some risk factors can be modified and/or eliminated.

- All body systems are affected to some extent by the aging process. Nevertheless, older adults can accept personal responsibility for avoiding many diseases and disabilities, minimizing risks, and maintaining physical and mental functioning.

- The majority of older adults live independently in community settings.

Tenets of Gerontological Nursing

Gerontological nursing practice involves interactive assessment and intervention that identifies and enhances an older adult's strengths and abilities to maximize well-being and quality of life. Guiding principles, or tenets for gerontological nursing include:

- Providing guidance and care to the older adult that respects human dignity and the uniqueness of the individual.

- Assisting the older adult to function at his or her highest level.

- Contributing to positive, realistic, and accurate perceptions of aging to society.

- Collaborating within health, social, political, cultural, and spiritual systems to eliminate the barriers and stereotyping of older adults.

- Assisting older adults in minimizing health risks includes recognition that:

  - Personal responsibility for one's own health status is central to healthy aging and instrumental in maintaining independence and control.

  - Physiologic changes and certain risk factors that occur with aging can be modified and individual adaptations made to prevent complications and decrease risks.

  - Physiologic, psychological, sociological, spiritual, cultural, and economic factors are interdependent forces that affect individual aging.

  - Stereotyping of older adults is a serious problem that contributes to societal fears of aging and negative practices such as age discrimination and elder abuse.

- Providing information, education, and resources to older adults and serving as advocates and change agents.

- Recognizing and addressing the frequently atypical response of older adults to disease and its treatment.

Trends in Population and Services

By examining the characteristics and needs of the aging population, balanced with an assessment of the current and projected changes in healthcare delivery systems, the gerontological nurse can determine appropriate nursing practice, research, educational, and administrative strategies.

Demographic Trends

The U.S. population of older adults (individuals >65 years of age) is growing rapidly. It is anticipated that between 1995 and 2030, this population will double from approximately 33.5 million to 69.4 million (Taeuber 1996). Adults aged 85 and greater are the fastest growing segment of the population. Their numbers are projected to increase from 3.6 million in 1995 to 8.5 million by 2030.

Included in this aging American population are growing numbers of older ethnic and racial minority populations. Minority populations represented approximately 15% of the elderly population in 1999; by 2030, that percentage is projected to rise to 25%. Between 1997 and 2030, the Hispanic population 65 and older is projected to increase by 368%, non-Hispanic blacks by 134%, non-Hispanic American Indians, Eskimos, and Aleuts by 159%, and non-Hispanic Asians and Pacific Islanders by 354% (AARP 1998).

Most older adults today are not severely limited in their activities of daily living (ADLs) despite living with chronic conditions. A majority of non-institutionalized persons 70 years of age and over report degenerative joint disease, one-third report hypertension, and approximately 11% have diabetes. Nearly 1 in 10 Americans has Alzheimer's disease or a related disorder. The average lifetime cost per patient for Alzheimer's disease is $174,000, making this the third most expensive disease in the United States after heart disease and cancer (Menzin, Lang, and Friedman 1999).

Despite their chronic conditions, less than 10% of non-institutionalized persons 70 years of age and over were unable to perform one or more ADLs (bathing, dressing, eating, toileting, transferring or ambulation) (National Center for 1996). Those who were older did tend to have more disability: Only 17% of individuals age 65 to 74 reported limitations in ADLs, compared with 27% percent of those 85 years of age and over.

Increasingly, older adults are engaging in preventive healthcare behaviors such as exercise. Unfortunately, the prevalence of leisure-time physical inactivity does increase with age, and is higher in African Americans and women (CDC 1999). Approximately one-third of those age 55 to 74 are inactive, and this increases to almost 50% of those age 75 or greater.

Service Trends

Almost all older adults in the United States have Medicare coverage, and approximately 12% of Medicare enrollees 65 years of age and older were in managed care plans in 1997. Individuals aged 65 and greater were consistently less likely to have a regular source of care than persons younger than 65 (National Center for Health Statistics 1995). Non-Hispanic black and Hispanic elderly individuals were less likely than non-Hispanic white older adults to have private insurance to supplement Medicare coverage. Financing of healthcare for older adults remains problematic.

Home healthcare continues to be an important segment in the healthcare industry and healthcare budgets. Among older adults living in the community, 1.75 million receive home healthcare services, including preventive, therapeutic, rehabilitative, restorative, and supportive care. Care providers include both formal (paid) caregivers and informal (unpaid) caregivers. Most care giving in the home (over 76%) is provided through informal support of family, friends, and neighbors (National Academy on an Aging Society 2000).

Additional services available to older adults who may be considered for nursing home placement include day care/respite programs, Programs for All-Inclusive Care for the Elderly (PACE 2000), and community-based programs targeting frail individuals. Community nursing organizations, house calls, and home rehabilitation augment these resources. Nursing home use increases dramatically with age and is close to 25% for white women 85 years of age or greater. Current estimates suggest that the chance of nursing home admission now approaches 43% for those who turned 65 in 1990. Of those who enter a nursing home, 55% will have a total lifetime use of 1 or more years, and for 21% percent, 5 years or more (Kemper and Murtaugh 1991).

Many older adults who would formerly have moved into nursing homes are being treated at home through home health agencies, or are turning to assisted living settings or other continuous care environments. Assisted living is a senior housing concept that combines residential housing with selected support services, commonly including meals, housekeeping, transportation, social activities, assistance with ADLs, and some nursing services (e.g., administration of medications). Resident acuity in assisted living is increasing as attempts are made to maintain older adults in these settings. Assisted living environments pose some challenges relative to financing care (the majority are private pay), staffing guidelines (few require licensed individuals on site), and restrictions on the ability to "age in place."

Hospitalization rates are higher for older adults, particularly those over 75 years of age. Approximately 10% of those age 45 to 74 were hospitalized compared with 20% of the those age 75 and greater (National Academy on an Aging Society 2000). Hospital stays for older adults are often complicated by underlying chronic conditions such as heart disease, degenerative joint disease, hearing and vision impairments, and dementias, all of which result in increased risk for complications and functional decline.

Gerontological Nursing Trends

The American Nurses Association continues to advocate and support the growing need for gerontological competence and expertise among nurses caring for older adults. Although the numbers of nurses certified in basic and advanced practice gerontological nursing has increased considerably over the years, additional nurses are needed to provide care, assist in transitions to new residential settings, and enhance quality of care to older adults in all settings. In addition to the role of care provider, the gerontological nurse is also responsible for educating and preparing other caregivers of older adults.

Approximately 15% of older adults experience a decline in cognitive function accompanying common physical problems. In the community, cognitive deficits are seen in 5% of those who are older than 65 years of age, and in 20% of those above 75 years of age. In the acute care setting, one-third to one-half of older adults have cognitive changes; more than 50% of those living in long-term care facilities are cognitively impaired (Kane, Ouslander, and Abrass 1999). Depression, delirium, paranoid states and other psychoses, anxiety, or amnestic syndromes are often associated with cognitive impairment. Consequently, psychogeriatric nursing practice is a rapidly developing specialty that addresses the mental health needs of older adults. Similarly, older adults with acquired immuno-deficiency syndrome (AIDS) are an additional cohort whose numbers are mounting. These individuals present with special challenges due to related disease changes superimposed on normal aging.

Gerontological nursing is one of the profession's most challenging practice areas. Gerontological nurses must continue to work with older adults in a variety of settings and meet the special needs of the increasing number of older adults, particularly those over 85 years of age, minorities, and those with decreased financial and social resources. Given the demographic shifts in the population and the use of high-end technology and life-sustaining services, the need for skilled gerontological nurses remains acute. Whether in the home, hospital, or various community and long-term care agencies, the older adult requires comprehensive care that focuses on individualized health promotion and disease prevention, ongoing assessment of functional and cognitive status, rapid identification of acute problems, rehabilitation and restorative care, ongoing education, and appropriate referrals.

Levels of Gerontological Nursing Practice

Basic Gerontological Nursing

The basic gerontological nurse is a licensed professional nurse who has demonstrated competency in gerontological nursing practice and practices in a variety of institutions, the home, and other community settings. The responsibilities of the gerontological nurse include direct care, management and development of professional and other nursing personnel, and evaluation of care and services for the older adult. All professional nurses practicing gerontological nursing are encouraged to acquire certification as a gerontological nurse.
    These nurses have the basic knowledge and skills to:

- Recognize the right of competent older adults to make their own care decisions and assist them in making informed choices.

- Establish a therapeutic relationship with the older adult to facilitate development of the plan of care, which may include family participation as needed.

- Use current gerontological standards to initiate, develop, and adapt the older adult's plan of care while involving the patient, family, and other providers as needed.

- Recognize age-related changes based on an understanding of physiologic, emotional, cultural, social, psychological, economic, and spiritual functioning.

- Collect data to determine health status and functional abilities to plan, implement, and evaluate care.

- Participate and collaborate with members of the interdisciplinary team.

- Participate with older adults, their families if needed, and other health professionals in ethical decision making that is centered on the older adult, empathetic and humane.

- Serve as an advocate for older adults and their families.

- Teach older adults and families about measures that promote, maintain, and restore health and functional performance; promote comfort; and foster independence and preserve dignity.

- Refer older adults to other professionals or community resources for assistance as necessary.

- Identify common chronic/acute physical and mental health processes and problems that affect older adults.

- Apply the existing body of knowledge in gerontology to nursing practice and intervention.

- Exercise accountability to older adults by protecting their rights and autonomy, recognizing and respecting their decisions about advance directives.

- Facilitate palliative care and comfort during the dying process to preserve dignity.

- Support the surviving spouse and family members, providing strength, comfort, and hope.

- Use the standards of gerontological nursing practice and collaborate with other healthcare professionals to improve the quality of care and quality of life of older adults.

- Engage in professional development through participation in continuing education, involvement in state and national professional organizations, and certification.

Advanced Practice Gerontological Nursing

The advanced practice gerontological nurse is a registered nurse (RN) who holds a master's, nursing doctorate, or higher degree, and demonstrates advanced knowledge and clinical expertise in the care of older adults. An advanced practice gerontological nurse is prepared to practice as a Clinical Nurse Specialist or Nurse Practitioner. The advanced practice gerontological nurse has the knowledge and skills to perform all aspects of basic gerontological nursing, and by virtue of graduate education has additional depth of knowledge and skills in theory, research, and practice. The roles of the advanced practice gerontological nurse include, but are not limited to, expert clinician, independent practitioner, educator, researcher, consultant, care manager, leader of interdisciplinary teams, and/or administrator. Advanced practice nurses practice within the scope of their state's nurse practice act. Advanced practice nurse who have fulfilled the requirements established by their state nurse practice act may be authorized to prescribe controlled substances or prescription drugs. Advanced practice gerontological nurses are encouraged to acquire certification.

The scope of practice in gerontological nursing is evolving and continually expanding as the science of nursing grows. The advanced practice gerontological nurse facilitates and supports health, wellness, healing and dying of older adults. The advanced practice nurse:

- Focuses on individuals, families, groups, communities or health-care systems.

- Is guided by theory and best evidence, and integrates creative and critical thinking.

- Demonstrates proficiency in influencing and/or developing health and social policy.

- Engages in the planning, implementation, and evaluation of health programs.

- Contributes to improved quality and cost-effective services.

- Generates, tests, and/or evaluates gerontological knowledge.

Gerontological nurses in advanced practice roles integrate relevant knowledge from nursing and other disciplines into their practice and participate in interdisciplinary relationships to create or influence the highest quality of care, the healthcare environment, and positive outcomes. Advanced practice gerontological nurses demonstrate knowledge, skill, forward thinking, and flexibility.

STANDARDS OF
CLINICAL GERONTOLOGICAL NURSING CARE

This section describes the competent level of clinical gerontological nursing care as demonstrated through assessment, diagnosis, outcome identification, planning, implementation, and evaluation. These processes encompass significant actions taken by gerontological nurses in providing care to older adults and form the foundation of clinical decision making. These standards apply to all gerontological nurses.

Standard I. Assessment

The gerontological nurse collects patient health data.

Rationale

Information obtained from older adults, families, significant others, and the interdisciplinary team and nursing knowledge is used to develop the comprehensive plan of care. These assessments must always be culturally and ethnically appropriate.

Measurement Criteria

1. The priority of data collection is determined by the older adult's immediate condition or needs.

2. The data may include, but are not limited to the following:

    a. Functional abilities (activities of daily living; ADLs)

    b. Physical, psychological, psychosocial, economic, cognitive, cultural, and spiritual status

    c. Environmental assessment, including safety issues and identification of available and accessible support systems and material resources

    d. Response to the aging process

    e. History of health patterns and illness(es)

f. Prescribed medication, self-medication, and complementary/integrative therapies and practices

g. Current self-care and health promotion activities

h. Past and current lifestyles

i. Individual coping patterns

j. Perception of and satisfaction with health status

k. Health beliefs, values, and practices

l. Knowledge of and receptivity to healthcare

m. Advance directives for healthcare

n. Strengths and competencies that can be used to promote health

3. Pertinent data are collected from multiple sources using various assessment techniques and standardized instruments as appropriate. Assessment data may be collected from the older adult and also significant others, formal and informal caregivers, members of the interdisciplinary care team, other healthcare providers, past and current health records, and community agencies.

4. The assessment process is systematic and ongoing.

5. Relevant data and risk factors are documented in a retrievable form, using a defined database when appropriate.

6. Health information must be maintained confidentially in all cases.

Standard II. Diagnosis

The gerontological nurse analyzes the assessment data in determining diagnoses.

Rationale

The gerontological nurse, either independently or in collaboration with interdisciplinary care providers, evaluates health assessment data to develop comprehensive diagnoses that guide interventions.

Measurement Criteria

1. Diagnoses are derived from assessment data.

2. Diagnoses and risk factors are validated with the older adult, family and significant others, as well as other healthcare providers when appropriate and possible.

3. Diagnoses identify actual or potential problems of the older adult that affect the individual's ability to:

    a. Maintain optimal health and well-being, prevent illness, prevent or minimize adverse effects of illness or functional decline, and experience a peaceful and dignified death.

    b. Adapt to limitations, functional impairments, or chronic conditions.

    c. Address physical, emotional, social, economic, cultural, environmental, and spiritual concerns.

    d. Manage symptoms and prevent or minimize the side effects or toxicities associated with pharmacologic interventions or other treatment regimens.

    e. Participate in therapeutic activities.

4. Diagnoses reflect the older adult's health knowledge and decision making ability.

5. Diagnoses are documented in a manner that facilitates the determination of expected outcomes and the development of a plan of care.

Standard III. Outcome Identification

The gerontological nurse identifies expected outcomes individualized to the older adult.

Rationale

The ultimate goals of providing gerontological nursing care are to influence health outcomes and improve or maintain the health status of the older adult. Outcomes often focus on maximizing the state of well-being, functional status, and quality of life.

Measurement Criteria

Expected outcomes:

1. Reflect the diagnoses.

2. Belong to the older adult (i.e., his or her goals) and are mutually formulated with the older adult, family or significant others, and interdisciplinary team members when possible.

3. Are culturally appropriate and realistic in relation to present and potential capabilities.

4. Are attainable in relation to resources available to the older adult and care setting.

5. Include a time frame for attainment.

6. Are identified with consideration of the associated benefits and costs.

7. Provide direction for continuity of care.

8. Are documented as measurable goals.

Standard IV. Planning

The gerontological nurse develops a plan of care that prescribes interventions to attain expected outcomes.

Rationale

A plan of care is used to structure and guide therapeutic interventions and achieve expected outcomes. It is developed in conjunction with the older adult, significant others, and interdisciplinary team members.

Measurement Criteria

1. The plan is individualized to the older adult's health status or needs and meets the following objectives:

   a. Identifies priorities of care in relation to expected outcomes.

   b. Identifies effective interventions to achieve outcomes.

c. Specifies interventions that reflect current gerontological nursing practice and research.

d. Includes, when appropriate, an educational program related to health maintenance and the older adult's health problems, treatment, and self-care activities.

e. Identifies environmental hazards and ways to address them, such as reducing exposure to high-frequency sounds, removing barriers to ambulation, and reducing stimuli to prevent or eliminate confusion.

f. Indicates responsibilities of the gerontological nurse and the older adult and may include responsibilities for interdisciplinary team members to carry out the plan of care.

g. Identifies a sequence of actions for achieving outcomes, as prioritized.

h. Gives directions for patient care activities delegated to other care providers.

i. Provides for appropriate referral and case management to ensure continuity of care.

j. Provides for quality of life as perceived by the older adult and, when appropriate, a good death.

k. Addresses the cultural, spiritual, therapeutic, preventive, restorative, and rehabilitative needs of the older adult.

l. Identifies the settings in which services may be safely and appropriately delivered.

m. Proposes alternatives for continuity of care for long-term needs.

n. Identifies resources required to accomplish the plan of care.

o. Includes a discharge plan, when appropriate.

2. The plan is developed in collaboration with the older adult, significant others, and interdisciplinary team members, when appropriate.

3. The plan is documented so that team members can review and modify it as necessary.

Standard V. Implementation

The gerontological nurse implements the interventions identified in the plan of care.

Rationale

The gerontological nurse uses a wide range of culturally competent interventions including health promotion, health maintenance, prevention of illness, health restoration, rehabilitation, and palliation. The gerontological nurse implements the plan of care in collaboration with the older adult and others.

Measurement Criteria

1. Interventions are selected on the basis of the needs, desires, and resources of the older adult and accepted nursing practice.

2. Interventions are selected and implemented according to the gerontological nurse's level of education, certification, and practice.

3. A therapeutic nurse–patient relationship is established and maintained.

4. Interventions are based on evidence-based practice, when available.

5. Interventions are implemented within the established plan of care and may include:

   • Facilitation of self-care and optimal functioning

   • Health promotion and maintenance

   • Disease prevention

   • Health teaching

   • Counseling

   • Psychobiological interventions

   • Consultation

   • Data collection and assessment

- Exploration of treatment choices, including integrated interventions/modalities such as nutrition, therapeutic touch, relaxation techniques, and exercise

- Palliative care for the chronically ill or dying older adult

- Referral to community resources

- Case management

- Evaluation and education of caregivers

6. Interventions are modified based on the continued assessment of the older adult's response to treatment and the clinical indicators of effectiveness.

7. Interventions are based on a knowledge of environmental effects on older adults.

8. Interventions are implemented in a safe, ethical, culturally competent and appropriate manner.

9. Interventions are documented.

Standard VI. Evaluation

The gerontological nurse evaluates the older adult's progress toward attainment of expected outcomes.

Rationale

Nursing practice is dynamic and evolving. The gerontological nurse continually evaluates the older adult's responses to treatment and interventions. Collection of new data, revision of the database, alteration of diagnoses, and modification of the plan of care are essential.

Measurement Criteria

1. Evaluation is systematic and ongoing, whether working with individuals, groups, or communities.

2. Older adults, families, and healthcare providers are involved in evaluation, as appropriate, to determine quality of life, satisfaction with care, and, to the degree possible, the benefits and costs associated with treatment.

3. The older adult's responses to treatment and interventions are documented.

4. The effectiveness of treatment and interventions are evaluated in relation to expected outcomes.

5. Ongoing assessment data are used to revise diagnoses, expected outcomes, and the plan of care as needed.

6. Revisions in diagnosis, expected outcomes, and the plan of care are reviewed with the older adult and caregiver(s) and documented to ensure continuity of care.

STANDARDS OF PROFESSIONAL GERONTOLOGICAL NURSING PERFORMANCE

This section on standards of professional performance describes a competent level of behavior in the professional role. All gerontological nurses are expected to engage in professional role activities appropriate to their education, position, and practice setting. Therefore, some standards or measurement criteria identify a broad range of activities that may demonstrate compliance with the standard.

Although this section describes the roles expected of all professional nurses, gerontological nursing encompasses many other responsibilities. Gerontological nurses should be self-directed and purposeful in seeking activities such as membership in professional organizations, certification in the specialty or advanced practice, and professional development through continuing education and further academic education, all of which are desirable methods of enhancing the gerontological nurse's professionalism.

Standard I. Quality of Care

The gerontological nurse systematically evaluates the quality of care and effectiveness of nursing practice.

Rationale

The dynamic nature and growing body of gerontological knowledge and research provide both the impetus and the means for gerontological nurses to improve the quality of patient care.

Measurement Criteria

The gerontological nurse:

1. Participates in quality of care and quality of life activities. Such activities may include:

    • Establishment of philosophy, goals, and standards of gerontological nursing services to create an environment that facilitates the provision of quality care and enhances the quality of life in both the community and all other care delivery environments.

- Identification of aspects of care important for quality monitoring such as cultural values, functional status, symptom management and control, health behaviors and practices, safety, satisfaction, and quality of life.

- Analysis of quality data to identify opportunities for improvement.

- Development of policies, procedures, and practice guidelines to improve quality of care and quality of life for the older adult.

- Identification of indicators used to monitor quality and effectiveness of care.

- Collection of data to monitor quality and effectiveness of care.

- Formulation of recommendations to improve nursing practice or patient outcomes.

- Implementation of activities to enhance the quality of nursing practice.

- Participation on interdisciplinary teams that evaluate clinical practice or health services.

2. Uses the results of quality activities to initiate changes in practice.

3. Uses the results of quality activities to initiate changes throughout the healthcare delivery system, as appropriate.

4. Integrates knowledge, research, and quality findings to provide guidance and leadership in the care of older adults.

Standard II. Performance Appraisal

The gerontological nurse evaluates his or her own nursing practice in relation to professional practice standards and relevant statutes and regulations.

Rationale

The gerontological nurse is accountable to the public for providing competent clinical care and has an inherent responsibility to practice according to standards established by the professional and regulatory bodies.

Measurement Criteria

The gerontological nurse:

1. Regularly engages in performance appraisal of his or her own clinical practice and clinical competence with peers or supervisors to identify areas of strength as well as areas for professional and practice development.

2. Seeks constructive feedback on practice and role performance from peers, professional colleagues, patients, and others.

3. Takes action to achieve goals identified during performance appraisal and peer review that result in changes in practice and role performance.

4. Participates in peer review activities as appropriate.

Standard III. Education

The gerontological nurse acquires and maintains current knowledge applicable to nursing practice.

Rationale

Scientific, cultural, societal, and political changes require a continuing commitment from the gerontological nurse to pursue knowledge to maintain competency, enhance nursing expertise, and advance the profession. Formal education, continuing education, certification, and experiential learning are some of the means for professional growth.

Measurement Criteria

The gerontological nurse:

1. Participates in ongoing educational activities to improve clinical knowledge, enhance role performance, and increase knowledge of professional nurses.

2. Seeks experiences and independent learning activities to maintain, refine, and develop clinical skills and knowledge.

3. Seeks knowledge and skills appropriate to the practice setting by participating in educational programs and activities, conferences, workshops, and interdisciplinary professional meetings.

Standard IV. Collegiality

The gerontological nurse contributes to the professional development of peers, colleagues, and others.

Rationale

The gerontological nurse is responsible for sharing knowledge, research, and clinical information with colleagues and others through formal and informal teaching methods and collaborative educational programs.

Measurement Criteria

The gerontological nurse:

1. Shares knowledge, research, clinical information, and skills with peers, colleagues, and others.

2. Helps others to identify teaching/learning needs related to clinical care, role performance, and professional development.

3. Provides peers with constructive feedback regarding their practice.

4. Contributes to an environment that is conducive to the clinical education of nursing students.

5. Participates in research and in the development of educational programs focusing on gerontological nursing, geriatrics, and gerontology for the older adult, care providers, and the community.

6. Participates in professional and community organizations.

Standard V. Ethics

The gerontological nurse's decisions and actions on behalf of older adults are determined in an ethical manner.

Rationale

The gerontological nurse is responsible for providing nursing services and healthcare that are responsive to the public's trust and the older adult's rights. Formal and informal care providers must also be prepared to provide the care needed and desired by the older adult and to render services in an appropriate setting.

Measurement Criteria

1. The gerontological nurse's practice is guided by the *Code of Ethics for Nurses with Interpretive Statements* (ANA 2001).

2. The gerontological nurse is concerned with issues such as informed consent, adherence to advance directives, emergency interventions, palliative care, pain management, need for self-determination, treatment termination, quality of life issues, chemical and physical restraints, confidentiality, surrogate decision making, complementary/integrative treatment modalities, fair distribution of resources, and economic decision making.

3. The gerontological nurse:

   - Maintains a therapeutic relationship with older adults and their significant others.

   - Maintains appropriate patient confidentiality within legal and regulatory parameters.

   - Functions as an advocate and assists older adults and their significant others, as appropriate, to advocate for themselves.

   - Respects the wishes of older adults without judgment and delivers care in a nondiscriminatory, culturally competent manner that is responsive to diversity.

   - Identifies ethical dilemmas that occur within the practice environment and seeks available resources to help formulate ethical decisions.

   - Delivers care in a manner that preserves the autonomy, dignity, and rights of the older adult.

   - Reports elder abuse, abuse of patient rights, incompetence, and unethical and illegal practices.

- Participates in informing older adults, families, and significant others of rights and responsibilities.

- Participates in obtaining the older adult's informed consent for procedures, treatment, and research, as appropriate.

- Informs older adults and their significant others, when appropriate, about the right to execute advance directives.

- Documents information about the interactions with older adults regarding rights and ethical issues, as appropriate.

Standard VI. Collaboration

The gerontological nurse collaborates with the older adult, the older adult's caregivers, and all members of the interdisciplinary team to provide comprehensive care.

Rationale

The complex nature of comprehensive care for older adults and their caregivers requires expertise from all members of the interdisciplinary team. Collaboration between healthcare consumers and providers is optimal for planning, implementing, and evaluating care. Communication among members of the interdisciplinary team provides a forum to evaluate the effectiveness of the plan of care and to utilize appropriate resources to achieve identified goals.

Measurement Criteria

The gerontological nurse:

1. Collaborates with older adults, caregivers, and members of the interdisciplinary team to formulate goals, a plan of care, and make decisions related to healthcare delivery.

2. Is knowledgeable about community resources.

3. Coordinates the care of the older adult, making referrals and providing for continuity of care, as needed.

4. Collaborates with other members of the interdisciplinary team in teaching, consultation, management, and research activities as appropriate.

5. Participates, when appropriate, in establishing clinical practice guidelines for interdisciplinary collaboration.

Standard VII. Research

The gerontological nurse interprets, applies, and evaluates research findings to inform and improve gerontological nursing practice.

Rationale

Gerontological nurses are responsible for improving current nursing practice and future healthcare for older adults by participating in the generation, testing, utilization, and evaluation of research findings. At the basic level of practice, the gerontological nurse participates in research studies, identifies clinical problems, and interprets and utilizes research findings to improve clinical care to older adults. At the advanced practice level, the gerontological nurse may be a full research participant in the generation, testing, utilization, critical evaluation, and dissemination of knowledge related to gerontological healthcare research.

Measurement Criteria

The gerontological nurse:

1. Utilizes substantiated research to provide best evidence for the basis of practice, as appropriate to his or her position, education, and practice environment.

2. Participates in research activities as appropriate to his or her position, education, and practice environment. Such activities may include the following:

   a. Conducting individual research or collaborating with a team of researchers.

   b. Identifying clinical problems suitable for gerontological nursing or interdisciplinary research.

   c. Participating in the development of the research plan.

   d. Participating in data collection and analysis.

   e. Communicating and disseminating findings.

f. Critiquing and evaluating research findings for application to practice.

g. Utilizing research findings to develop policies, procedures, and guidelines for patient care.

h. Consulting with other researchers.

i. Providing gerontological research references/resources in the practice setting.

3. Protects the rights and welfare of individuals who participate as subjects in research activities.

VIII. Resource Utilization

The gerontological nurse considers factors related to safety, effectiveness, and cost in planning and delivering patient care.

Rationale

The older adult is entitled to healthcare that is safe, ethical, effective, acceptable, and affordable. Treatment decisions consider quality of care and appropriate utilization of resources.

Measurement Criteria

The gerontological nurse:

1. Reviews the benefits and cost of treatment options with the older adult, significant others, and other providers, as appropriate.

2. Helps the older adult and significant others identify and secure appropriate and affordable quality services available to address health-related needs.

3. Assigns tasks and delegates and supervises care based on the needs of the older adult and on the knowledge and skill of the selected provider.

4. Is cognizant of state and federal regulations and the implications of those regulations related to the delivery of care to older adults.

GLOSSARY

Activities of daily living (ADLs)—Daily activities related to personal care (dressing, bathing, toileting, grooming, transferring, ambulation, and eating).

Advance directives—The older adult's expression of preferences for future care.

Advanced practice gerontological nurse—A nurse practitioner and/or clinical specialist who holds at least a master's degree in nursing, has advanced clinical experience, and demonstrates extensive knowledge, competence, and skill in the care of older adults.

Assessment—A systematic, dynamic process by which the nurse, through interaction with the older adult, significant others, and healthcare providers, collects and analyzes data about the older adult. Data may include the following dimensions: physical, psychological sociocultural, spiritual, cognitive, functional abilities, developmental, economic, and lifestyle.

Assisted living—A residential or facility-based program that provides, in return for payment, housing and supportive services, supervision, personalized assistance, health-related services, or a combination thereof to meet the needs of residents who are unable to perform, or need assistance in performing, the activities of daily living (ADLs) or instrumental activities of daily living. Care is provided in a way that promotes optimum dignity and independence for the residents.

Caregivers—Individuals who provide care to older adults. Formal caregivers include those individuals who are paid to provide care services. Informal caregivers include those individuals who are not paid.

Case management—The assessment, planning, coordination, and evaluation of the effectiveness of health-promoting services for an individual.

Certification—The formal process by which clinical competence is validated by a certifying organization in the specialty area of practice.

Code of Ethics for Nurses with Interpretive Statements **(Code of Ethics for Nurses)** — A set of moral rules with interpretive statements that establishes the ethical imperatives that should shape nursing practice. The Code describes the ethical duties of the nurse and establishes the professional parameters for all interactions and interventions on behalf of patients, their families and communities. The Code also enumerates the nurse's duties to self and to the profession.

Collaboration — An interactive process whereby nurses and other healthcare professionals within an organization and/or the larger community work together, within their respective scopes of practice, for the benefit of the older adult. Healthcare providers who successfully collaborate demonstrate a shared philosophy of care for the older adult and mutual respect for each other.

Complementary care — Complementary care is a broad domain of healing resources that encompasses all health systems, modalities, and practices and their accompanying theories and beliefs, other than those considered as conventional. Complementary care includes all practices that are used to prevent or treat illness or promote health and well-being.

Criteria — Relevant, measurable indicators of the standards of clinical nursing practice.

Diagnosis — A clinical judgment about the patient's response to actual or potential health conditions or needs. Diagnoses are the basis for a care plan.

Evaluation — The process of determining both the older adult's progress toward expected outcomes and the effectiveness of nursing care.

Functional status — A multidimensional concept that characterizes the older adult's ability to perform activities related to the activities of daily living (ADLs), social interactions, occupational functioning, and use of leisure time.

Gerontological — Related to the aging process.

Gerontology — The study of all aspects of the aging process, including physical, psychosocial, spiritual, economic, and disease related.

Health—The positive state of full functioning in relation to one's capabilities and lifestyle, not merely the absence of disease or infirmity.

Implementation—Intervention, delegation, or coordination by the older adult, significant others, or healthcare providers to carry out the plan of care.

Interdisciplinary team—An interactive team of professionals from different disciplines who work together to define the situation for each patient and to respond to all of the patient's needs under a plan developed by the entire group.

Managed care—A broad continuum of entities, from the simple requirement of prior authorization for a service in an indemnity health insurance plan to the assumption of all legal, financial, and organizational risks, for the provision of a set of comprehensive benefits to a defined population. Also, the management of healthcare clinical services supplied by groups of providers with the aims of cost effectiveness, quality, and accessibility.

Nurse Practice Act—State laws that define the parameters of practice for registered nurses.

Outcomes—Measurable, expected, client-focused goals that focus on maximizing the older adult's state of well-being, functional status, and quality of life.

PACE—An acronym for the *Program for All-inclusive Care of the Elderly*, a program that provides for older adults so that they are able to stay in their own homes with sufficient support.

Palliative care—Care intended to lessen the violence of disease by controlling pain and making the process of dying as dignified and comfortable as possible.

Peer review—The process by which registered nurses actively engaged in the practice of nursing appraise the quality of care in a given situation in accordance with established standards of practice.

Professional code—Statement of ethical guidelines for nursing behavior that serves as a framework for decision making.

Psychogeriatric—Relating to mental healthcare of the older adult.

Registered nurse—An individual educationally prepared in nursing and licensed by the state board of nursing to practice in that state. Registered nurses may qualify for specialty practice at two levels, basic and advanced. These levels are differentiated by educational preparation, professional experience, type of practice, and certification.

Rehabilitation—An interdisciplinary process that focuses on returning the older adult to their highest possible level of psychological and physical health and functional ability.

Restorative care—A philosophy of care that focuses on regaining and maintaining the highest possible functional level of the older adult.

Scope of practice—A range of nursing functions that are differentiated according to the level of practice, the ole of the nurse, and the work setting. The parameters are determined by each state's nurse practice act, professional code of ethics, and nursing practice standards, as well as each individual's personal competency to perform particular activities or functions.

Standards of nursing practice—Statements describing a level of care of performance, common to the profession of nursing, by which the quality of nursing practice can be judged. They include activities related to assessment, diagnosis, outcome identification, planning, implementation, evaluation, quality of care, performance appraisal, education, collegiality, ethics, collaboration, research, and resource utilization.

Theory—The coherent set of hypothetical, conceptual, and pragmatic principles forming the general frame of reference for a field of inquiry. The body of generalizations or principles developed in association with practice in a field of activity and forming its content as an intellectual discipline.

APPENDIX

HISTORY OF GERONTOLOGICAL NURSING SCOPE AND STANDARDS

1966   ANA Division of Geriatric Nursing Practice formed

1976   Division of Geriatric Nursing Practice name changed to Division on Gerontological Nursing Practice to reflect the emphasis on health and aging

1976   *Standards of Gerontological Nursing Practice* first published

1981   Statement on the *Scope of Gerontological Nursing Practice* published

1984   ANA Council on Gerontological Nursing formed, aimed at improving the quality of care and the quality of life for aging persons

1987   *Standards and Scope of Gerontological Nursing Practice* published

1994   ANA restructured to combine councils; the Council for Community, Primary, and Long Term Care was developed to address the healthcare needs of those in the community, individuals who were well, and those who needed institutional long-term care

1995   *Scope and Standards of Gerontological Nursing Practice*, revised, published

2001   *Scope and Standards of Gerontological Nursing Practice, 2nd Edition*, revised, published

REFERENCES

American Association of Retired Persons (AARP). 1998. *A Profile of Older Americans*. Washington, D.C.: AARP.

American Nurses Association (ANA). 2001. *Code of Ethics for Nurses with Interpretive Statements*. Washington, DC: American Nurses Publishing.

— — —. 1998. *Standards of Clinical Nursing Practice, 2nd ed*. Washington, DC: American Nurses Publishing.

— — —. 1995. *Scope and Standards of Gerontological Nursing Practice*. Washington, DC: American Nurses Publishing.

— — —. 1987. *Standards and Scope of Gerontological Nursing Practice*. Kansas City, MO.: ANA.

— — —. 1981. *A Statement on the Scope of Gerontological Nursing Practice*. Kansas City, MO: ANA.

— — —. 1976. *Standards of Gerontological Nursing Practice*. Kansas City, MO: ANA.

Centers for Disease Control and Prevention (CDC). 1999. Surveillance for selected public health indicators affecting older adults— United States. *Morbidity and Mortality Weekly Report: CDC Surveillance Summaries* 48(SS-8). Available from http://www.cdc.gov/mmwr/indss_99.html; INTERNET.

Kane, R., J. G. Ouslander, and I. B. Abrass. 1999. *Essentials of Clinical Geriatrics*. New York: McGraw-Hill.

Kemper, P., and C. N. Murtaugh. 1991. Lifetime use of nursing home care. *New England Journal of Medicine* 324: 595–600.

Menzin, J., K. Lang, and M. Friedman. 1999. The economic cost of Alzheimer's disease to a state program. *Neurology* 52 (6 suppl 2): A8.

National Academy on an Aging Society. 2000. *Care Giving: Helping the Elderly with Activity Limitations.* (May) Issue #7.

National Center for Health Statistics (NCHS).1996. *Data File Documentation, National Health Interview Survey of Disability, Phase I, 1994.* Hyattsville, Md.: National Center for Health Statistics, Centers for Disease Control and Prevention (CDC).

— — —. 1998. *Data File Documentation, National Health Interview Second Supplement on Aging, 1994.* Hyattsville, Md.: National Center for Health Statistics, Centers for Disease Control and Prevention (CDC).

Programs of All-inclusive Care for the Elderly (PACE) 2000. Title 42 — Public Health Chapter IV. Subchapter E, Part 460. Healthcare Financing Administration, Department of Health and Human Services. [42 CFR Ch. IV (10-1-00 Edition).] Available from http://www.access.gpo.gov/nara/cfr/cfrhtml_00/Title_42/42cfr460_00.html; INTERNET.

Rowe, J. W., and Kahn, R. L. 1998. *Successful Aging.* New York: Pantheon.

Taeuber, C. 1996. *Sixty-five Plus in America.* Current Population Reports. Special Studies. Publication P23-173RV. Washington D.C.: U.S. Department of Commerce, Economics and Statistics Administration, Bureau of the Census.

INDEX

An index entry followed by [2001] indicates content from the previous edition *Scope and Standards of Gerontological Nursing Practice*, which is reproduced as Appendix A

A

AACN. *See* American Association of Colleges of Nursing
Activities of daily living (ADLs), 81
[2001]
Adult-gerontological population focus, 13
Advanced practice gerontological nurse practitioners, 11, 13
advocacy role, 7, 20, 54
assessment, 29
collaboration, 46
collegiality, 45
consultation, 37
coordination of care, 35
defined, 55
diagnosis, 30
education, 43–44
ethics, 48
evaluation, 39
health teaching and health promotion, 36
leadership, 53
need for APRNs with gerontology specialty, 17
outcomes identification, 31
plan implementation responsibilities, 34
planning responsibilities, 32–33
prescriptive authority and treatment, 38
professional practice evaluation, 42
quality of practice, 41
regulation model, 13
research, 49–50
resource utilization, 51
standards of practice, 29–39
standards of professional performance, 41–54
Advocacy in gerontological nursing, 7, 20, 54

Age-appropriate care in gerontological nursing, 15, 17, 27
developmental and cognitive issues and, 1, 8, 30, 36, 38
See also Cultural competence and sensitivity
Aging. *See also* Older adults
assumptions, 1–2
of population, 2–3
as public health issue, 23
physiology, 25
[2001], 77–81
Almshouses as early norm of care, 4–5
American Association of Colleges of Nursing (AACN), 6f, 6, 12, 19
American Geriatrics Society, 19
American Nurses Association (ANA), 4–5, 6f, 14
American Nurses Credentialing Center (ANCC), 14
American Nurses Foundation (ANF), 14
Assessment in gerontological nursing, 9
defined, 55
in nursing process, 8, 25, 27
in measurement criteria, 30, 33, 34, 39
standard of practice, 29
[2001], 87–88
Assessment data
in diagnosis, 30
in evaluation, 39
Assisted living, 8, 13
defined, 55
[2001], 82
Atlantic Philanthropies, 11, 14

B

Bahr, Rose Therese, 6f
Building Academic Gerontology Nursing Capacity (BAGNC), 11

C

Care and caring in gerontological
    nursing, 3–4
  legal standard of, 28
  palliative and hospice, 22
  See also Coordination of care; Planning
    and plan of care
Caregivers in gerontological nursing
  defined, 55
  family and informal, 4, 19
  See also Healthcare providers
Centers of Gerontological Nursing
    Excellence, 11
Certification in gerontological nursing,
    10, 13, 16
  alternate examination, 17
  competencies for various, 17–19
  defined, 55
Chronic illness in older adults, 3–4
  end of life issues in, 21
  multiple conditions in, 2, 9
  palliative care and, 22
  uniqueness of, 25
Clinical education opportunities in
    gerontological nursing, 13–14
Clinical practice development, 11
Coalition for Geriatric Nursing
    Organizations, 22
Code of Ethics for Nurses, 21, 47
  defined, 55
  See also Ethics
Cognitive and developmental issues in
    older adults, 1, 15, 30, 36, 38
Collaboration in gerontological nursing,
    1, 28, 34
  defined, 55
  standard of professional performance,
    46
  [2001], 100–101
Collegiality in gerontological nursing
  standard of professional performance,
    45
  [2001], 98
Community-based care in geronto-
    logical nursing, 3–4, 13
Competency in gerontological nursing,
    12, 17, 19

competencies and certification, 17–19
  defined, 55
  educators and, 16
  Nurse Competency on Aging, 14
Confidentiality, 47
  HIPPA and, 21
Consensus Model for APRN Regulation,
    13
Consultation in gerontological nursing
  standard of practice, 37
Continuing education in gerontological
    nursing, 14, 18
Continuity of care, 30, 31, 32, 46
  defined, 55
Coordination of care in gerontological
    nursing, 51, 52
  standard of practice, 35
Cost controls and issues in gerontological
    nursing, 38
  outcomes identification and, 31
  resource utilization and, 51
Council on Gerontological Nursing, 65f
Crane, Carolyn, 4
Cultural competency and sensitivity in
    gerontological nursing, 1, 2, 3, 17
  HRSA initiative, 15
  nurse adeptness in, 27
  in measurement criteria, 29, 31, 36, 42,
    47
Culture change and nursing home care,
    21–22

D

Data (defined), 56
Data collection and analysis in geronto-
    logical nursing
  in measurement criteria, 29, 30, 31, 35,
    37, 39, 49
  See also Assessment data
Demographic trends in aging, 2–3
Developmental and cognitive issues in
    older adults, 1, 8, 30, 36, 38
Diagnosis in gerontological nursing
  assessment data and, 30
  defined, 55
  in measurement criteria, 31, 32, 34, 38,
    39

Nursing science development, 11
  See also Research

O
Old Americans Act, 5
Older adults and gerontological nursing,
  1, 7–9, 28
  characteristics, 1–3
  heterogeneity of, 2, 25
  See also Aging
Outcomes evaluation in gerontological
  nursing
  standard of practice, 39
Outcomes identification in gerontological
  nursing
  in nursing process, 8, 25, 27
  standard of practice, 31
  [2001], 89–90

P
Palliative and hospice care in gerontological nursing, 22
Paraprofessionals, 18
Patient (defined), 57
Patient safety issues in gerontological
  nursing, 9
  advocacy and, 54
  legal obligations of nurses, 21
  resource utilization and, 51
  workforce and workplace aspects of,
  24
Peer review and relationships in gerontological nursing, 42, 45, 49
  peer review (defined), 57
Performance appraisal [2001]
  standard of professional performance,
  96–97
Person-centered approach gerontological nursing, 7, 32, 54
Personal liability, 21
Pharmacology and pharmaceuticals.
  See Prescriptive authority and
  treatment
Physiology of aging, 25
  [2001], 78–79
Pioneer Network, 21–22
Plan (defined), 57

Plan of care, 22, 34
  coordination of, 35
  See also Planning
Planning
  in nursing process, 8, 25, 27
  standard of practice, 32
  [2001], 90–91
Polypharmacy in older adults, 9
Population, aging of, 2–3
Practice settings for gerontological
  nursing, 7–8
Prescriptive authority and treatment in
  gerontological nursing
  drug interactions in older adults, 9
  mental health and, 15
  standard of practice, 38
Primary care settings and clinical
  education opportunities, 13
Professional associations, 24
Professional development, 14–16
Professional liability, 21
Professional performance. See Standards
  of professional performance
Professional practice evaluation, 42
Promotive practice in gerontological
  nursing, 3, 7, 16, 20, 24
  See also Health teaching and health
  promotion
Psychogeriatric nursing practice [2001],
  83
  See also Geropsychiatric nursing
  practice
Public health aspect of aging, 23
Public service, 8

Q
Quality of care in gerontological nursing,
  1, 25
  defined, 58
  [2001], 95–96
Quality of life, 1, 2, 3, 25
  palliative care and, 22
  [2001], 95–96
Quality of practice in gerontological
  nursing
  standard of professional performance,
  41